Easy Nursing English

看単！
かんたん

Ian Willey
Gerardine McCrohan
芝田征二
著

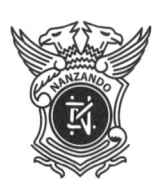

南山堂

執筆者

イアン・ウィリー   Ian Willey
香川大学 大学教育基盤センター 准教授
Associate Professor, Higher Education Center, Kagawa University

ジェラディーン・マクラハン   Gerardine McCrohan
香川大学 大学教育基盤センター 准教授
Associate Professor, Higher Education Center, Kagawa University

芝田 征二   Seiji Shibata
香川大学 名誉教授
Professor Emeritus, Kagawa University

協力者

キシ ケイコ イマイ   Keiko Imai Kishi, BS, MNSc, DNSc
元 佐久大学 教授 / 元 香川大学 医学部 看護学科 教授
Former Professor, Saku University / Former Professor, School of Nursing, Faculty of Medicine, Kagawa University / RN

川﨑 緑   Midori Kawasaki, Master of Welfare Sociology
元 明治国際医療大学 看護学部 教授
Former Professor, School of Nursing Science, Meiji University of Integrative Medicine / RN

波多江 優   Suguru Hatae, MNS
JA神奈川県厚生連 相模原協同病院 外来・患者総合支援センター 看護師 / がん看護専門看護師
RN, Patient Support Center, Sagamihara Kyodo Hospital / Certified Nurse Specialist in Cancer Nursing

安田壽賀子   Sugako Yasuda
香川大学 医学部附属病院 元 看護師長 / 元 香川大学 医学部 看護学科 臨床准教授
RN, Former Head Nurse, Department of Nursing, Kagawa University Hospital
Former Clinical Associate Professor, School of Nursing, Faculty of Medicine, Kagawa University

大島由紀江   Yukie Oshima, ADN
香川大学 医学部附属病院 看護師長 / 皮膚・排泄ケア認定看護師
RN, Head Nurse, Department of Nursing, Kagawa University Hospital / WOC Certified Nurse

今出 政代   Masayo Imade, ADN
香川大学 医学部附属病院 看護師 / 緩和ケア認定看護師
RN, Department of Nursing, Kagawa University Hospital / Palliative Care Certified Nurse

上原 正宏   Masahiro Uehara, MS
香川大学 医学部 小児科 客員研究員
Visiting Researcher (Department of Pediatrics), Faculty of Medicine, Kagawa University

上原 典子   Noriko Uehara, M Pol

推薦のことば

看護英語テキスト"看単！ Easy Nursing English"の推薦のことばを依頼されることは大変光栄なことだと思います．推薦にあたって述べたいのは以下のことです．

最近，国際化ブームにのって，日本中の英語教育方法が変化していくなか，看護分野においても海外ボランティア，JICA などで英語が共通語として使われる国で活躍する看護職者が増加してきました．そこでの日常臨床活動において問題となるのは，現地の援助として問題解決をしたくても，医学用語，患者との会話など，他の国の医療従業者とのコミュニケーションが英語でうまくとれないことです．日本国内においても同様な問題がおきていて，それは日本に来ている日本語を話さない外国人研修者，その家族，外国人労働者などが日本の医療施設，サービスを使う機会が増えてきたからです．それに対応して大学制の看護教育においては看護英語という科目を提供し，国際間のコミュニケーションの改善をはかろうとしています．

一方，看護英語教育をする教師も日本人英語教師の他，母国語が英語である英語教師が採用されるようになりました．当テキストの執筆者も，日本語しか話さない看護学生を対象に，現場で看護英語を使って英会話ができるための教育を行ってきた経験から，このテキスト作成に臨みました．

現在，電子辞書として，看護大辞典，医学大辞典がでまわっている時代に，書籍としての看護英語テキストの特典は何でしょうか．本書は，英語に関して初心者の学生，看護職者に必要最低限の医学用語・単語 500 語以上を網羅し，日常の臨床でおこる会話の事例を状況ごとに提供し，演習はクロスワーズパズルと取り組むようなゲーム感覚で楽しみながら，やさしい問題から難しい問題にという進み方をしています．演習の最後は自分で新しい医学用語・単語のスペリングができるように工夫されています．本書の Index は辞書として使えるので，これを持っていれば，いつでもどこでも勉強ができます．教師のためには，授業でこのテキストを使うときの提案例があり，授業に取り組みやすくなっています．一般に学生の自己学習の集中力の限界は 30 分から 45 分といわれているので，1 週間に 1 章をこなせば，一学期の終わりには，看護英語を使って必要最低限の英会話ができるようになるはずです．勉強するのが楽しいというのは大切なことです．

以上の理由で，私はこの看護英語テキストを看護学生，国際協力に関わっている看護職者，看護英語担当教師，および英語が苦手であると思っている医療従業者にぜひおすすめしたいのです．

2009 年 1 月

キシ ケイコ イマイ　看護科学博士

About this Book

There are plenty of Nursing English vocabulary books on the market. Our goal was to produce a workbook that presents basic vocabulary useful for nurse-to-patient communication, with lots of sample sentences and exercises to help the reader to remember these terms, and how to use them. We believe that this workbook can be used both in a classroom and as a self-study book for students and practicing nurses.

In writing it, we tried to:

1) **present basic Nursing English vocabulary**, 20~25 words or phrases per chapter. Due to space constraints some important words had to be left out. Professional or "medical" terms are marked by ⓜ. All unmarked words are standard or common usages.

2) **use American English terms and spellings**. This is mainly due to the fact that Japanese students are more familiar with American English, and to keep this book short and simple we did not include British usages.

3) **show sentences as they would occur in a Japanese hospital or clinic**. This has not always been possible, as many words are not normally used in nurse-to-patient communication. Some sentences may sound artificial. And some may sound as though they belong in an English-speaking context. As long as an example sentence helps the reader to remember a word, and how it can be used, then we believe that it is a good sentence.

We are not nurses. For this reason we relied on the help of nursing professionals and educators while planning and writing this book, and their guidance has given it professional authenticity. We give special thanks to the collaborators on page ii. Any flaws that remain are our own responsibility.

We believe that English is useful for nurses in Japan. English ability can help nurses to communicate with a broad range of patients, refine their clinical knowledge, and open doors to career opportunities. It can help you to become someone whom patients, other nurses, and doctors can depend upon. If this book helps you in any small way, then it has done its work.

Ian Willey
Gerardine McCrohan
Seiji Shibata

Takamatsu, Japan
January, 2009

看護英語の本は数多く出版されています．そのなかで私たちは，語彙を覚えて使うための例文や練習問題を豊富に盛り込み，看護師と患者さんとのコミュニケーションに役立つ基礎的な語彙を収載したワークブックを作ることを目指しました．本書は看護学生・看護師の方々のための授業テキストとして，または自主学習教材としても利用していただけるものと自負しています．

本書を書くにあたっては，次のようなことに配慮しました．

1） 基礎的な語彙を選んで収載した．各章20～25の英単語・英文を掲載．誌面の都合上，一部割愛せざるを得なかった用語もある．専門用語には ⑩ 印を付した．この印がない語は一般的な語である．

2） 米国英語の用語・スペリングを用いた．これは，日本の学生の皆さんが米国英語に慣れ親しんでいること，そして，英国英語の用例併記を避けて簡潔な内容にしたかったことによる．

3） 日本の病院や診療所で出会う文章を収載．看護師と患者さんとのコミュニケーションで通常使われない語も多いため，すべてを実際に出会う文章にすることはできなかった．なかには不自然な文章，英語的な言い回しの文章もあるかもしれない．しかし，読者の方々が語彙を覚え，それがどのように使われるのかを示す一助となるという点では，こうした文章にも意味があると思われる．

私たちは看護師ではないため，本書の企画制作を通じて，看護師と看護分野の教官に協力を仰ぎ，そのおかげで，本書の内容はより確実なものとなりました．先のページに掲げた協力者の方々に心より感謝申し上げます．

英語は日本の看護師の皆さんにきっと役立つはずだと信じています．患者さんと広くコミュニケーションをとるために，臨床知識を磨くために，キャリアアップの扉を開くために，英語の能力が助けになります．また，患者さん・周りの看護師・医師に頼りにされることにもなります．もし，少しでもあなたのお役に立てたなら，この本は役割を果たしたと言えるでしょう．

イアン・ウィリー

ジェラディーン・マクラハン

芝　田　征　二

高松にて

2009年1月

Table of Contents

── Part One   Basic medical words   基本医学用語

Section I: People, places and things in a hospital/clinic   病院のスタッフ・施設・物品

Chapter 1. Hospital departments and associated doctors   診療科と専門医 3
Chapter 2. Healthcare personnel, patients, and other people   医療従事者と患者およびその関係者 7
Chapter 3. Medical supplies and equipment   医療用品と器具 11
Chapter 4. Medication and treatment   薬剤と治療 15

Section II: Anatomical words   身体用語

Chapter 5. External body   外部器官 19
Chapter 6. Internal body I   内部器官 I 23
Chapter 7. Internal body II   内部器官 II 27
Chapter 8. Musculoskeletal system   筋骨格系 31

Section III: Illnesses and emergencies   疾患と救急

Chapter 9. Illnesses and conditions I   病気と症状 I 35
Chapter 10. Illnesses and conditions II   病気と症状 II 39
Chapter 11. Children's and women's illnesses and conditions   小児・婦人科の疾患と症状 43
Chapter 12. Injuries and emergencies   外傷と救急 47

Table of Contents

Part Two　Basic communication　基本的なコミュニケーション表現

Section IV: Nurse-to-patient communication　患者とのコミュニケーション

Chapter 13.　Common complaints　主訴 53

Chapter 14.　Taking a patient's history　病歴の聴取 57

Chapter 15.　Giving instructions during an examination　検査時の助言 61

Chapter 16.　Common questions from foreign patients　外国人患者がよく問う質問 65

Section V: Communication and encouragement　コミュニケーションと励ましの言葉

Chapter 17.　Daily routine communication　看護師の日常会話 69

Chapter 18.　Words of encouragement　励ましの言葉 73

Supplement (Teacher's manual)

Extension task 78

Answers 80

Index 116

Part One
Basic medical words
基本医学用語

Section I   People, places and things in a hospital/clinic   病院のスタッフ・施設・物品

- **Chapter 1** Hospital departments and associated doctors   診療科と専門医
- **Chapter 2** Healthcare personnel, patients, and other people   医療従事者と患者およびその関係者
- **Chapter 3** Medical supplies and equipment   医療用品と器具
- **Chapter 4** Medication and treatment   薬剤と治療

Section II   Anatomical words   身体用語

- **Chapter 5** External body   外部器官
- **Chapter 6** Internal body I   内部器官 I
- **Chapter 7** Internal body II   内部器官 II
- **Chapter 8** Musculoskeletal system   筋骨格系

Section III   Illnesses and emergencies   疾患と救急

- **Chapter 9** Illnesses and conditions I   病気と症状 I
- **Chapter 10** Illnesses and conditions II   病気と症状 II
- **Chapter 11** Children's and women's illnesses and conditions   小児・婦人科の疾患と症状
- **Chapter 12** Injuries and emergencies   外傷と救急

Section I   People, places and things in a hospital/clinic

Chapter 7

1. Hospital departments and associated doctors
診療科と専門医

	Department	Doctor	日本語
1.	anesthesiology	anesthesiologist	麻酔科（麻酔科医）
2.	cardiology	cardiologist	循環器内科（循環器内科医）
3.	dentistry	dentist	歯科（歯科医）
4.	dermatology	dermatologist; skin doctor	皮膚科（皮膚科医）
5.	endocrinology	endocrinologist	内分泌科（内分泌科医）
6.	gastroenterology	gastroenterologist	消化器内科（消化器内科医）
7.	geriatrics	geriatrician	老年内科（老年内科医）
8.	gynecology ☺	gynecologist	婦人科（婦人科医）
9.	internal medicine	internist; physician	内科（内科医）
10.	neurology	neurologist	神経内科（神経内科医）
11.	neurosurgery	neurosurgeon	脳神経外科（脳神経外科医）
12.	obstetrics	obstetrician	産科（産科医）
13.	oncology	oncologist	腫瘍内科（腫瘍内科医）
14.	ophthalmology	ophthalmologist ⓜ; eye doctor	眼科（眼科医）
15.	orthopedics	orthopedist	整形外科（整形外科医）
16.	otorhinolaryngology; otolaryngology	otorhinolaryngologist ⓜ; otolaryngologist; ENT doctor (ENT=Ear, Nose and Throat)	耳鼻咽喉科（耳鼻咽喉科医）
17.	pediatrics	pediatrician; children's doctor	小児科（小児科医）
18.	plastic surgery; reconstructive surgery	plastic surgeon	形成外科（形成外科医）
19.	psychiatrics	psychiatrist	精神科（精神科医）
20.	pulmonology	pulmonologist	呼吸器内科（呼吸器内科医）
21.	radiology	radiologist	放射線科（放射線科医）
22.	urology	urologist	泌尿器科（泌尿器科医）

☺ An obstetrician/gynecologist is called an OB-GYN ([óu-bíː-ʤín], [óu-bíː-ʤíː-wái-én]) doctor.

ⓜ medical word

Part One Basic medical words

Exercise 1. Match the English word on the left with a Japanese word on the right.

1.	oncology	a.	内分泌科
2.	neurology	b.	腫瘍内科
3.	geriatrics	c.	形成外科
4.	gastroenterology	d.	消化器内科
5.	ophthalmology	e.	整形外科
6.	pulmonology	f.	神経内科
7.	cardiology	g.	老年内科
8.	orthopedics	h.	眼科
9.	plastic surgery	i.	循環器内科
10.	endocrinology	j.	呼吸器内科

1.____ 2.____ 3.____ 4.____ 5.____ 6.____ 7.____ 8.____ 9.____ 10.____

Exercise 2. Read the following sentences and <u>underline</u> the correct word in parentheses ( ).
The first one is done for you.

1. My five-year-old son has just been admitted to the (<u>pediatrics</u> / pediatrician) department.

2. Ms. Chun works in the (psychiatrics / psychiatrist) department.

3. A (gynecology / gynecologist) treats only women.

4. For your X-ray you will have to go to (radiology / radiologist).

5. Dr. Harris is an (otorhinolaryngology / otorhinolaryngologist).

6. An (obstetrics / obstetrician) delivers babies.

7. Dr. Sekiguchi is a renowned (neurosurgery / neurosurgeon).

8. An (anesthesiology / anesthesiologist) will put you to sleep before the operation.

9. (Reconstructive surgery / Reconstructive surgeon) is on the second floor.

10. My husband is seeing a (urology / urologist) tomorrow.

4

Section I People, places and things in a hospital/clinic   Chapter 1

Exercise 3. Complete these sentences with words in the box below. Each word is used only once.

1. If you have a toothache, you should see a _____ promptly.

2. Yuji likes children and hopes to become a _____ nurse.

3. A _____ is concerned with treating elderly people.

4. To have your eyes checked, you should go to the _____ department.

5. Many people have the flu now so _____ is busy.

6. Mr. Yamamoto spent two weeks in the _____ department with a broken leg.

7. You have a bad sunburn. You need to see a _____.

8. Japanese hospitals need more _____.

9. Patients with cancer are treated in _____.

10. If your ear is in pain you should see an _____.

```
oncology      geriatrics     pediatrics      obstetricians        dermatologist
orthopedics   geriatrician   internal medicine                    ophthalmology
dentist       dermatology    otorhinolaryngologist                neurology
```

◇ **Dialogue**

Nurse: Can I help you?
Patient: Yes. Can you tell me how to get to dermatology?
Nurse: Sure. Just go down this corridor, and you'll see the elevator on your right. Dermatology is on the third floor. You'll see the reception window as soon as you get off.
Patient: Thank you. I don't have an appointment. Is there usually a long wait?
Nurse: You won't have to wait too long. About 30 minutes.
Patient: Oh. Well, I hope there are newspapers or magazines to read.
Nurse: There are. But I'm afraid they're all in Japanese!

Part One   Basic medical words

Self-study sheet

Write the correct English words in the blanks. Learn them by heart!

1.	麻酔科		麻酔科医	
2.	循環器内科		循環器内科医	
3.	歯科		歯科医	
4.	皮膚科		皮膚科医	
5.	内分泌科		内分泌科医	
6.	消化器内科		消化器内科医	
7.	老年内科		老年内科医	
8.	婦人科		婦人科医	
9.	内科		内科医	
10.	神経内科		神経内科医	
11.	脳神経外科		脳神経外科医	
12.	産科		産科医	
13.	腫瘍内科		腫瘍内科医	
14.	眼科		眼科医	
15.	整形外科		整形外科医	
16.	耳鼻咽喉科		耳鼻咽喉科医	
17.	小児科		小児科医	
18.	形成外科		形成外科医	
19.	精神科		精神科医	
20.	呼吸器内科		呼吸器内科医	
21.	放射線科		放射線科医	
22.	泌尿器科		泌尿器科医	

Good work! ☺

Section I People, places and things in a hospital/clinic

Chapter 2

2. Healthcare personnel, patients, and other people
医療従事者と患者およびその関係者

Vocabulary	日本語
1. head nurse	病棟師長
2. surgical nurse; scrub nurse	手術室看護師
3. community health nurse	保健師
4. midwife	助産師
5. registered nurse (RN)	看護師
6. physician; doctor; practitioner	医師
7. attending physician	主治医
8. clinical resident, resident	研修医
9. pharmacist	薬剤師
10. X-ray technician	放射線技師
11. dietitian; nutritionist	栄養士
12. clinical psychologist	臨床心理士
13. physical therapist	理学療法士
14. dental hygienist	歯科衛生士
15. EMT (Emergency Medical Technician)	救急救命士
16. receptionist	受付係
17. cashier	会計窓口係
18. care worker; care giver	介護福祉士
19. inpatient	入院患者
20. outpatient	外来患者
21. guardian	保護者
22. visitor	面会者

Part One Basic medical words

Exercise 1. Match the English word on the left with a Japanese word on the right.

1. physician
2. clinical resident
3. pharmacist
4. X-ray technician
5. clinical psychologist
6. inpatient
7. outpatient
8. community health nurse
9. attending physician
10. receptionist

a. 主治医
b. 受付係
c. 保健師
d. 医師
e. 研修医
f. 薬剤師
g. 臨床心理士
h. 外来患者
i. 放射線技師
j. 入院患者

1.____ 2.____ 3.____ 4.____ 5.____ 6.____ 7.____ 8.____ 9.____ 10.____

Exercise 2. Read the following sentences and underline the correct word in parentheses ( ).

1. (An X-ray technician / A pharmacist) works in radiology.

2. Make an appointment with the (receptionist / cashier) at the front desk.

3. If you stay overnight in a hospital you are an (inpatient / outpatient).

4. A (nutritionist / dental hygienist) can help you choose healthy foods.

5. A (care giver / midwife) helps with the delivery of babies.

6. A (head nurse / surgical nurse) works in an operating room.

7. (Visitors / Outpatients) may come during the visiting hours.

8. (EMTs / Attending physicians) rushed to the accident site in an ambulance.

9. A (pharmacist / practitioner) can fill your prescription.

10. A (physical therapist / clinical psychologist) can help you learn to walk again.

Section I People, places and things in a hospital/clinic   Chapter 2

Exercise 3. Complete these sentences with words in the box below. Each word is used only once.

1. You should pay the _____ on the first floor.

2. _____ should be quiet so as not to disturb patients' rest.

3. A _____ will clean and polish your teeth.

4. Please speak to a _____ about your diet.

5. Hospitals need more _____ these days.

6. The _____ will help you to rebuild your muscle strength.

7. Please give this prescription to the _____.

8. More _____ are needed to take care of elderly people in their homes.

9. Are you this child's _____?

10. My name is Yuko Miyatake. I am the _____ of this section.

```
    guardian      head nurse     receptionist    registered nurses    dietitian
    physical therapist      EMT         pharmacist          visitors
    cashier          midwife        dental hygienist      care workers
```

◇ Dialogue

Patient: What do I do now?
Nurse: First you'll have to pay. Give this file to the cashier on the first floor. You'll have to show your insurance card, too.
Patient: Will my prescription be filled there?
Nurse: You'll have to go to the pharmacy for that. There's one in front of this hospital. Just give the prescription to the receptionist. You won't have to wait long.
Patient: Will they be able to explain the medicine to me?
Nurse: I think so. Be sure to ask if there is anything you don't understand.
Patient: Thank you for your help.
Nurse: It's my pleasure.

Part One Basic medical words

Self-study sheet

Write the correct English words in the blanks. Learn them by heart!

1. 病棟師長	
2. 手術室看護師	
3. 保健師	
4. 助産師	
5. 看護師	
6. 医師	
7. 主治医	
8. 研修医	
9. 薬剤師	
10. 放射線技師	
11. 栄養士	
12. 臨床心理士	
13. 理学療法士	
14. 歯科衛生士	
15. 救急救命士	
16. 受付係	
17. 会計窓口係	
18. 介護福祉士	
19. 入院患者	
20. 外来患者	
21. 保護者	
22. 面会者	

Nice job! ☺

Section I People, places and things in a hospital/clinic

3. Medical supplies and equipment
医療用品と器具

Vocabulary	日本語
1. bandage	包帯
2. gauze	ガーゼ
3. disinfectant	消毒液
4. crutch, crutches (pl)	松葉杖
5. sutures; stitches	縫合
6. cast	ギプス
7. sling	三角巾
8. wheelchair	車椅子
9. walker	歩行器
10. stretcher	ストレッチャー
11. stethoscope	聴診器
12. sphygmomanometer[m], manometer; blood pressure gauge	血圧計
13. tongue depressor	舌圧子
14. hearing aid	補聴器
15. endoscope	内視鏡
16. gastroscope	胃カメラ
17. needle	針
18. syringe	注射器
19. inhaler	吸入器
20. respirator	人工呼吸器
21. IV[☺] pole; IV stand	点滴棒，点滴スタンド
22. bedpan	便器
23. washbasin; sink	洗面器
24. scale (weight scale; height scale)	体重計，身長計
25. treatment table	処置台

☺ IV = intravenous

[m] medical word

Part One   Basic medical words

Exercise 1.   Match the English word on the left with a Japanese word on the right.

1. sling
2. disinfectant
3. crutches
4. gauze
5. height scale
6. IV pole
7. stethoscope
8. endoscope
9. syringe
10. needle

a. 針
b. 内視鏡
c. 点滴棒
d. 聴診器
e. 消毒液
f. 注射器
g. ガーゼ
h. 身長計
i. 三角巾
j. 松葉杖

1.____   2.____   3.____   4.____   5.____   6.____   7.____   8.____   9.____   10.____

Exercise 2.   Read the following sentences and underline the correct word in parentheses (   ).

1. We put your husband on a (respirator / endoscope) because he can't breathe on his own.

2. Please stand on the (cast / scale) so we can see how much you weigh.

3. Please sit in the (wheelchair / inhaler) so we can take you to radiology.

4. I want to change the (bandage / needle) on your wound.

5. Your arm is broken so you will need a (wheelchair / cast) for about a month.

6. This is a deep cut. You will need some (disinfectant / stitches) to close it.

7. When the doctor puts the (gastroscope / tongue depressor) in your mouth, please say "ah."

8. You're making progress. You can walk well using a (walker / sling) now.

9. If you can't hear me clearly, please put in your (syringe / hearing aid).

10. Please lie on the (scale / treatment table) so the doctor can examine you.

12

Section I   People, places and things in a hospital/clinic   Chapter 3

Exercise 3. Complete these sentences with words in the box below. Each word is used only once.

1. We'll use a _____ to take you to the operating room.

2. You cannot take a shower because you need to keep your _____ dry.

3. The doctor will use a _____ to listen to your breathing.

4. Nurse, the _____ from my IV is hurting a little.

5. You have five _____ keeping the wound closed.

6. This _____ will help you control your asthma symptoms.

7. You can wash your face in the _____ but you can't have a bath yet.

8. Please use the _____ when you need to go to the toilet.

9. I'll use a _____ to check your blood pressure. Roll up your sleeve, please.

10. The doctor will use a _____ to look inside your stomach.

cast	washbasin	stitches	stethoscope	syringe
needle	inhaler	respirator	blood pressure gauge	
wheelchair	bedpan	gastroscope	stretcher	

◇ Dialogue

Patient: How long will I have to keep this cast on?
Nurse: The doctor said you'll have to wait at least one more week.
Patient: How about these stitches above my eye?
Nurse: Those should stay in for a few more days.
Patient: That's a relief. They're starting to itch. If only I could take this cast off sooner...
Nurse: I'm afraid you must wait until the bone has properly healed. It won't be too much longer.
Patient: I know. I just can't wait.
Nurse: To walk again?
Patient: To play rugby again!
Nurse: Well, you should take it easy for a while before playing any sports again.

Part One Basic medical words

Self-study sheet

Write the correct English words in the blanks. Learn them by heart!

1. 包帯	
2. ガーゼ	
3. 消毒液	
4. 松葉杖	
5. 縫合	
6. ギプス	
7. 三角巾	
8. 車椅子	
9. 歩行器	
10. ストレッチャー	
11. 聴診器	
12. 血圧計	
13. 舌圧子	
14. 補聴器	
15. 内視鏡	
16. 胃カメラ	
17. 針	
18. 注射器	
19. 吸入器	
20. 人工呼吸器	
21. 点滴棒	
22. 便器	
23. 洗面器	
24. 体重計	
25. 処置台	

Outstanding! ☺

Section I People, places and things in a hospital/clinic

Chapter 4

4. Medication and treatment
薬剤と治療

Vocabulary	日本語
1. pill	錠剤(じょうざい)
2. liquid medicine	水薬(みずぐすり)
3. powdered medicine	散剤(さんざい)
4. suppository	坐薬(ざやく)
5. antibiotic, antibiotics	抗菌薬(こうきんやく),抗生物質(こうせいぶっしつ)
6. analgesic[m], painkiller	鎮痛剤(ちんつうざい)
7. cough suppressant; cough medicine	鎮咳剤(ちんがいざい)
8. herbal medicine	漢方薬(かんぽうやく)
9. sleeping pill	睡眠剤(すいみんざい)
10. laxative	下剤(げざい)
11. gargle; mouthwash	含そう剤(がんそうざい),うがい薬(ぐすり)
12. ointment; salve	軟膏(なんこう)
13. over-the-counter medicine (OTC medicine)	市販薬(しはんやく)
14. prescription, to prescribe (v)	処方箋(しょほうせん),処方(しょほう)する
15. contraceptive	避妊薬(ひにんやく)
16. dosage, dose	投薬量(とうやくりょう)
17. directions	使用説明(しようせつめい)
18. once a day (*quaque die*; *q.d.*)	1日(にち)1回(かい)
19. after meals (*post cibum*; *p.c.*)	食後(しょくご)
20. at bedtime (*hora somni*; *h.s.*)	就寝時前(しゅうしんじまえ),眠前(みんぜん)
21. IV☺ drip	点滴静脈注射(てんてきじょうみゃくちゅうしゃ)
22. blood transfusion	輸血(ゆけつ)
23. dialysis	人工透析(じんこうとうせき)
24. organ transplantation	臓器移植(ぞうきいしょく)
25. surgery; operation	手術(しゅじゅつ)

☺ IV = <u>i</u>ntra<u>v</u>enous
[m] medical word

15

Part One   Basic medical words

Exercise 1. Match the English word on the left with a Japanese word on the right.

1. suppository
2. cough medicine
3. laxative
4. liquid medicine
5. herbal medicine
6. ointment
7. once a day
8. blood transfusion
9. organ transplantation
10. surgery

a. 臓器移植
b. 手術
c. １日１回
d. 軟膏
e. 坐薬
f. 鎮咳剤
g. 輸血
h. 下剤
i. 漢方薬
j. 水薬

1.____ 2.____ 3.____ 4.____ 5.____ 6.____ 7.____ 8.____ 9.____ 10.____

Exercise 2. Read the following sentences and underline the correct word in parentheses ( ).

1. I have a terrible headache. Can I have a (painkiller / laxative) please?

2. Please apply this (gargle / ointment) to the burn twice a day.

3. Aspirin is a common (over-the-counter medicine / antibiotic) in many countries.

4. This (sleeping pill / cough medicine) will help you to sleep.

5. You've lost a lot of blood so you will need (surgery / a blood transfusion).

6. Take your (pill / prescription) to the pharmacy on the first floor.

7. Please follow the (prescription / directions) carefully.

8. Take this sleeping pill (after meals / at bedtime).

9. The (dosage / contraceptive) is different depending on the size and age of the patient.

10. You have a three-day supply of these (antibiotics / contraceptives).

Section I People, places and things in a hospital/clinic   Chapter 4

Exercise 3. Complete these sentences with words in the box below. Each word is used only once.

1. Saachi needs _____ regularly because her kidneys have failed.

2. Take the small white _____ twice a day.

3. You will have an _____ in your arm when you wake up from the operation.

4. In many countries _____ is becoming more common. You can get a new kidney, heart or liver if you need one.

5. You will need an _____ to remove your appendix.

6. To prevent colds it is good to use a _____ often.

7. Take the antibiotic three times a day _____.

8. This _____ will help you go to the toilet more easily.

9. An oral _____ is an alternative to a condom.

10. Take this _____ if your headache returns.

```
pill         organ transplantation    IV drip       suppository    after meals
contraceptive    dialysis             directions    painkiller     laxative
gargle           operation            over-the-counter medicine
```

◇ Dialogue

Patient: I don't understand the directions for this medicine. Could you explain them to me?

Nurse: I'd be happy to. These large round pills are antibiotics. You should take them three times a day after each meal.

Patient: I see.

Nurse: These small oval-shaped pills are painkillers. Take them only when you have a bad headache.

Patient: Can I take them on an empty stomach?

Nurse: It's best not to. Please take them with food. Now, this powdered medicine will relieve your cold symptoms. Take it in the morning and evening, after breakfast and dinner.

Patient: This is complicated. I hope I can remember!

Nurse: Just don't lose these directions! I'm sure you'll be fine.

Part One Basic medical words

Self-study sheet

Write the correct English words in the blanks. Learn them by heart!

1. 錠剤	
2. 水薬	
3. 散剤	
4. 坐薬	
5. 抗生物質	
6. 鎮痛剤	
7. 鎮咳剤	
8. 漢方薬	
9. 睡眠剤	
10. 下剤	
11. うがい薬	
12. 軟膏	
13. 市販薬	
14. 処方箋	
15. 避妊薬	
16. 投薬量	
17. 使用説明	
18. 1日1回	
19. 食後	
20. 就寝時前	
21. 点滴静脈注射	
22. 輸血	
23. 人工透析	
24. 臓器移植	
25. 手術	

So far, so good! ☻

5. External body
外部器官

Vocabulary	日本語
1. forehead	前額部
2. cheek	頬部, 頬
3. jaw	あご
4. chin	頤
5. neck	頚部, 首
6. shoulder	肩
7. axilla[m]; armpit	腋窩
8. chest	胸部
9. breast	乳房
10. nipple	乳頭
11. upper arm	上腕部
12. forearm	前腕部
13. elbow	肘部, 肘
14. abdomen	腹部
15. skin	皮膚
16. wrist	手関節, 手首
17. hip	股関節部, 腰周り
18. buttocks	殿部, 尻
19. genitals	生殖器
20. thigh	大腿部
21. knee	膝
22. ankle	足関節
23. heel	踵部
24. hallux[m]; toe	つま先
25. nail	爪

[m] medical word

Part One Basic medical words

Exercise 1. Match the English word on the left with a Japanese word on the right.

1. forehead
2. chin
3. armpit
4. knee
5. forearm
6. abdomen
7. wrist
8. thigh
9. ankle
10. nail

a. 足関節
b. 前額部
c. 大腿部
d. 爪
e. 前腕部
f. 頤
g. 手関節
h. 腋窩
i. 膝
j. 腹部

1.____ 2.____ 3.____ 4.____ 5.____ 6.____ 7.____ 8.____ 9.____ 10.____

Exercise 2. Unscramble these words. Write the Japanese on the second line. The first one is done for you.

	English	日本語
1. kcne	neck	頚部
2. redluosh		
3. sbtutcok		
4. preup mar		
5. weblo		
6. eto		
7. slagetin		
8. nisk		
9. iph		
10. pinlep		

Section II Anatomical words   Chapter 5

Exercise 3. Complete these sentences with words from the box below. Each word is used only once.

1. He was punched in the face and broke his _____.

2. Laina fell and twisted her _____. Now she can't walk very well.

3. You have very pale _____. Be sure to wear sunscreen in the summer.

4. Are you _____-feeding your baby?

5. Please put the thermometer under your arm, in your _____.

6. Lie on your back. The doctor will listen to your _____.

7. You have dislocated your _____, and will have to use a sling for a while.

8. Mr. Fernandez has a burning pain in his _____ from his ulcer.

9. Oh my, her _____ are red. Your daughter has a high fever.

10. Jeong Soon needed three stitches in her _____ after stepping on broken glass.

| heel | shoulder | skin | breast | abdomen | jaw |
| cheeks | ankle | chest | armpit | forearm | buttocks |

◇ Dialogue

Mr. Hossain: I would like to see the doctor about a pain in my shoulder. It has become severe.
Nurse: That's not good. Do you have your insurance booklet?
Mr. Hossain: I just started a new job, and have not received one yet. But I am covered by the national system.
Nurse: Well, can you give us the phone number of your place of employment?
Mr. Hossain: Actually, I do not know. Can I tell the office at work, and have them call you?
Nurse: That would be fine, but please have them call as soon as possible. We're open until 12:00 and then close for lunch. Afternoon hours are from 2:30 to 6:00.
Mr. Hossain: Thank you. I appreciate it.
Nurse: It's my pleasure.

Part One Basic medical words

Self-study sheet

Write the correct English words in the blanks. Learn them by heart!

1. 前額部	
2. 頬	
3. あご	
4. 頤	
5. 首	
6. 肩	
7. 腋窩	
8. 胸部	
9. 乳房	
10. 乳頭	
11. 上腕部	
12. 前腕部	
13. 肘部	
14. 腹部	
15. 皮膚	
16. 手首	
17. 股関節部	
18. 殿部	
19. 生殖器	
20. 大腿部	
21. 膝	
22. 足関節	
23. 踵部	
24. つま先	
25. 爪	

You're going strong now! ☺

Section II Anatomical words

Chapter 6

6. Internal body I
Nervous, Sensory, Respiratory & Digestive system
内部器官 I ― 脳神経系, 感覚系, 呼吸器系, 消化器系

	Vocabulary	日本語
1.	brain	脳 (のう)
2.	spinal cord	脊髄 (せきずい)
3.	nerve	神経 (しんけい)
4.	tympanic membrane(m); eardrum	鼓膜 (こまく)
5.	nasal cavity	鼻腔 (びくう)
6.	throat	咽喉 (いんこう)
7.	pharynx	咽頭 (いんとう)
8.	larynx; voice box	喉頭 (こうとう)
9.	tonsil	扁桃腺 (へんとうせん)
10.	trachea; windpipe	気管 (きかん)
11.	lung	肺 (はい)
12.	diaphragm	横隔膜 (おうかくまく)
13.	tongue	舌 (した)
14.	gingiva(m); gum	歯肉 (しにく)
15.	esophagus	食道 (しょくどう)
16.	stomach	胃 (い)
17.	small intestine	小腸 (しょうちょう)
18.	large intestine	大腸 (だいちょう)
19.	colon	結腸 (けっちょう)
20.	vermiform appendix(m), appendix	虫垂 (ちゅうすい)
21.	rectum	直腸 (ちょくちょう)
22.	liver	肝臓 (かんぞう)
23.	gallbladder	胆嚢 (たんのう)
24.	pancreas	膵臓 (すいぞう)
25.	feces; stool	便 (べん)

(m) medical word

23

Part One Basic medical words

Exercise 1. Match the English word on the left with a Japanese word on the right.

1. brain   a. 膵臓
2. nerve   b. 小腸
3. tonsil   c. 脳
4. larynx   d. 横隔膜
5. trachea   e. 気管
6. diaphragm   f. 歯肉
7. gum   g. 扁桃腺
8. small intestine   h. 神経
9. colon   i. 結腸
10. pancreas   j. 喉頭

1.____ 2.____ 3.____ 4.____ 5.____ 6.____ 7.____ 8.____ 9.____ 10.____

Exercise 2. Fill in the missing words or letters to complete these terms. Then write the Japanese in the second space.

日本語

1. _____ cord   _____

2. nasal _____   _____

3. _____ membrane   _____

4. voice _____   _____

5. _____ bladder   _____

6. large _____   _____

7. vermiform _____   _____

8. _____ pipe   _____

9. _____ phagus   _____

10. rect_____   _____

Section II Anatomical words   Chapter 6

Exercise 3. Complete these sentences with words in the box below. Each word is used only once.

1. Boris drinks too much alcohol and has _____ damage now.

2. Your _____ is red. It looks very sore.

3. While eating an apple, Susan accidentally bit her _____.

4. Pharyngitis is a painful inflammation of the _____.

5. You will need to bring a urine and _____ sample for your health examination.

6. Petra injured her _____ and is paralyzed from the waist down.

7. Cigarette smoking can cause _____ cancer.

8. I have a _____ ache after eating oysters.

9. Too much meat in one's diet can lead to _____ cancer.

10. Bicycle helmets can prevent _____ injury.

| lung | stomach | voice box | tongue | stool | spinal cord |
| liver | throat | gallbladder | pharynx | colon | brain |

◇ Dialogue

Nurse: This paper gives information about your gastroscopic examination. Please don't eat anything after 9:00 pm the night before. And don't drink anything after midnight.

Patient: Can I brush my teeth in the morning?

Nurse: You can, but don't swallow any water. Be sure also to wear loose-fitting clothes.

Patient: Can I drive here?

Nurse: It's better to walk, or have someone drive you. The anesthesia will make driving or riding a bicycle dangerous.

Patient: Will it be painful? I'm really worried about this.

Nurse: You'll feel some discomfort, but it won't be as bad as you think. This is the best way to find out what's happening in your stomach.

Part One Basic medical words

Self-study sheet

Write the correct English words in the blanks. Learn them by heart!

1. 脳	
2. 脊髄	
3. 神経	
4. 鼓膜	
5. 鼻腔	
6. 咽喉	
7. 咽頭	
8. 喉頭	
9. 扁桃腺	
10. 気管	
11. 肺	
12. 横隔膜	
13. 舌	
14. 歯肉	
15. 食道	
16. 胃	
17. 小腸	
18. 大腸	
19. 結腸	
20. 虫垂	
21. 直腸	
22. 肝臓	
23. 胆嚢	
24. 膵臓	
25. 便	

Keep at it! ☺

7. Internal body II
Circulatory, Blood and Immune, Endocrine, Reproductive & Urogenital system
内部器官 II — 循環器系，血液・免疫系，内分泌系，泌尿・生殖器系

Vocabulary	日本語
1. heart	心臓 (しんぞう)
2. artery	動脈 (どうみゃく)
3. vein	静脈 (じょうみゃく)
4. valve	弁 (べん)
5. spleen	脾臓 (ひぞう)
6. plasma	血漿 (けっしょう)
7. leukocyte[m]; white blood cell	白血球 (はっけっきゅう)
8. erythrocyte[m]; red blood cell	赤血球 (せっけっきゅう)
9. bone marrow	骨髄 (こつずい)
10. lymph node	リンパ節 (せつ)
11. thyroid gland	甲状腺 (こうじょうせん)
12. penis	陰茎 (いんけい)
13. testicle	精巣 (せいそう)
14. sperm	精子 (せいし)
15. prostate	前立腺 (ぜんりつせん)
16. vagina	膣 (ちつ)
17. cervix	子宮頚管 (しきゅうけいかん)
18. uterus; womb	子宮 (しきゅう)
19. ovary	卵巣 (らんそう)
20. placenta	胎盤 (たいばん)
21. kidney	腎臓 (じんぞう)
22. ureter	尿管 (にょうかん)
23. urinary bladder, bladder	膀胱 (ぼうこう)
24. urine	尿 (にょう)
25. urethra	尿道 (にょうどう)

[m] medical word

Part One   Basic medical words

Exercise 1.   Match the English word on the left with a Japanese word on the right.

1. artery
2. valve
3. plasma
4. placenta
5. urethra
6. penis
7. testicle
8. vagina
9. ovary
10. urine

a. 卵巣
b. 弁
c. 膣
d. 動脈
e. 尿道
f. 胎盤
g. 精巣
h. 尿
i. 血漿
j. 陰茎

1.____   2.____   3.____   4.____   5.____   6.____   7.____   8.____   9.____   10.____

Exercise 2.   Fill in the missing words or letters to complete these terms. Then write the Japanese in the second space.

日本語

1. bone _____   _____

2. prost_____   _____

3. _____ node   _____

4. _____ gland   _____

5. _____ bladder   _____

6. erythro_____   _____

7. white blood _____   _____

8. uter_____   _____

9. _____ney   _____

10. cerv_____   _____

Section II Anatomical words   Chapter 7

Exercise 3. Complete these sentences with words in the box below. Each word is used only once.

1. Nurse, I'm having trouble passing _____.

2. The nurse had difficulty finding my _____. I should lose weight.

3. The common word for "erythrocyte" is _____.

4. A high _____ count may indicate infection.

5. You have a growth on the wall of your _____.

6. _____ cancer develops most frequently in men over fifty.

7. The _____ disposes of old red blood cells.

8. The _____ is a tube that carries urine from the kidney to the bladder.

9. My husband has a low _____ count.

10. Serge suffered severe chest pains and was diagnosed as having had a _____ attack.

ureter	sperm	spleen	white blood cell
vein	red blood cell	kidney	heart
urine	uterus	cervix	prostate

◇ **Dialogue**

Woman: Can you explain the results of my son's blood test? I still don't understand.

Nurse: Well, this number is your son's white blood cell count. It's very high, which shows your son still has an infection—a urinary tract infection.

Woman: And why did the doctor circle this number?

Nurse: This is the amount of iron in your son's blood. It's very low. He appears to be anemic.

Woman: The doctor did mention that. That's why my son has to take that brown medicine.

Nurse: That's right. Iron is needed to bring oxygen to the lungs, which may explain your son's fatigue.

Woman: Does he need to eat more iron-rich foods, like liver?

Nurse: That will help, but he'll also have to take iron supplements.

Woman: This sounds serious. But at least I know now. Thank you.

Part One Basic medical words

Self-study sheet

Write the correct English words in the blanks. Learn them by heart!

1. 心臓	
2. 動脈	
3. 静脈	
4. 弁	
5. 脾臓	
6. 血漿	
7. 白血球	
8. 赤血球	
9. 骨髄	
10. リンパ節	
11. 甲状腺	
12. 陰茎	
13. 精巣	
14. 精子	
15. 前立腺	
16. 膣	
17. 子宮頸管	
18. 子宮	
19. 卵巣	
20. 胎盤	
21. 腎臓	
22. 尿管	
23. 膀胱	
24. 尿	
25. 尿道	

Perfect! ☺

Section II Anatomical words

Chapter 8

8. Musculoskeletal system
筋骨格系

Vocabulary	日本語
1. muscle	筋肉 (きんにく)
2. cartilage	軟骨 (なんこつ)
3. tendon	腱 (けん)
4. ligament	靭帯 (じんたい)
5. joint	関節 (かんせつ)
6. bone	骨 (ほね)
7. cranium(m); skull	頭蓋骨 (ずがいこつ)
8. maxilla(m); upper jaw	上顎骨 (じょうがくこつ)
9. mandible(m); lower jaw	下顎骨 (かがくこつ)
10. clavicle(m); collar bone	鎖骨 (さこつ)
11. scapula(m); shoulder blade	肩甲骨 (けんこうこつ)
12. spine; backbone	脊椎 (せきつい), 脊柱 (せきちゅう)
13. vertebra(m), vertebrae (pl)	脊椎骨 (せきついこつ)
14. sternum(m); breastbone	胸骨 (きょうこつ)
15. rib	肋骨 (ろっこつ)
16. pelvis	骨盤 (こつばん)
17. coccyx(m); tail bone	尾骨 (びこつ)
18. humerus(m)	上腕骨 (じょうわんこつ)
19. ulna(m)	尺骨 (しゃっこつ)
20. radius(m)	橈骨 (とうこつ)
21. carpus(m); wrist bone	手根骨 (しゅこんこつ)
22. patella(m); kneecap	膝蓋骨 (しつがいこつ)
23. femur(m); thigh bone	大腿骨 (だいたいこつ)
24. fibula(m)	腓骨 (ひこつ)
25. tibia(m); shin bone	脛骨 (けいこつ)

(m) medical word

31

Part One Basic medical words

Exercise 1. Match the English word on the left with a Japanese word on the right.

1.	bone	a.	腓骨
2.	tendon	b.	靭帯
3.	joint	c.	腱
4.	vertebra	d.	脊椎骨
5.	rib	e.	軟骨
6.	pelvis	f.	骨盤
7.	fibula	g.	骨
8.	radius	h.	橈骨
9.	cartilage	i.	肋骨
10.	ligament	j.	関節

1.____ 2.____ 3.____ 4.____ 5.____ 6.____ 7.____ 8.____ 9.____ 10.____

Exercise 2. Complete the table. The first one is done for you.

	Medical word	Common word	日本語
1.	cranium	skull	頭蓋骨
2.	maxilla		
3.		lower jaw	
4.			鎖骨
5.		shoulder blade	
6.	spine		
7.			胸骨
8.		kneecap	
9.	carpus		
10.			脛骨
11.			大腿骨

Section II   Anatomical words   Chapter 8

Exercise 3. Complete these sentences with words in the box below. Each word is used only once.

1. Mr. Park was hit in the head and his _____ was fractured.

2. The _____ is the strongest bone in the human body.

3. Katarina broke her _____ last year, and sometimes she feels pain in her shoulder.

4. I was hit in the chest playing football and cracked two of my _____.

5. Miss Inoue broke her _____ in her right forearm.

6. Mr. Wolki fractured his _____ just above his elbow.

7. I'm afraid a _____ in your wrist is torn. You'll need surgery to repair it.

8. Too much exercise can damage your _____.

9. Ms. Taladoc feels pain in her _____ when she sits down.

10. Fortunately, your grandmother didn't break her _____ when she fell.

```
femur      ligament    skull       ulna       ribs      collar bone
humerus    bone        tail bone   pelvis     muscles   joint
```

◇ Dialogue

Nurse: Hello, Mr. Gommlich. How is your knee today?

Mr. Gommlich: It is still throbbing, but not as badly as yesterday.

Nurse: Hmm. Your torn ligament was successfully repaired, but it will take time to heal.

Mr. Gommlich: My leg bone hurts as well, right here.

Nurse: That's from the screw drilled into your tibia. You'll have to use crutches for the next week so that you don't put your full weight on your knee.

Mr. Gommlich: When does physical therapy begin?

Nurse: Actually, I'm here to take you to therapy now. Are you ready?

Mr. Gommlich: Ready as I will ever be!

Nurse: That's the spirit! Before long you'll be walking again.

Part One   Basic medical words

Self-study sheet

Write the correct English words in the blanks. Learn them by heart!

1. 筋肉	
2. 軟骨	
3. 腱	
4. 靱帯	
5. 関節	
6. 骨	
7. 頭蓋骨	
8. 上顎骨	
9. 下顎骨	
10. 鎖骨	
11. 肩甲骨	
12. 脊椎	
13. 脊椎骨	
14. 胸骨	
15. 肋骨	
16. 骨盤	
17. 尾骨	
18. 上腕骨	
19. 尺骨	
20. 橈骨	
21. 手根骨	
22. 膝蓋骨	
23. 大腿骨	
24. 腓骨	
25. 脛骨	

Keep going! ☺

Section III Illnesses and emergencies

Chapter 9

9. Illnesses and conditions Ⅰ
Nervous; Ear, Nose, Throat and Eye; Respiratory; Digestive; Blood and Immune; and Endocrine systems
病気と症状Ⅰ — 脳神経系，耳鼻咽喉系，呼吸器系，消化器系，血液・免疫系，内分泌系

Vocabulary	日本語
1. cerebrovascular accident[m] (CVA); stroke	脳卒中 (のうそっちゅう)
2. migraine	片頭痛 (へんずつう)
3. meningitis	髄膜炎 (ずいまくえん)
4. pollinosis[m]; hay fever	花粉症 (かふんしょう)
5. otitis media[m]; middle ear infection	中耳炎 (ちゅうじえん)
6. blindness	視覚障害 (しかくしょうがい)
7. deafness	聴覚障害 (ちょうかくしょうがい)
8. muteness	言語・音声障害 (げんご・おんせいしょうがい)
9. common cold	かぜ，感冒 (かんぼう)
10. laryngitis	喉頭炎 (こうとうえん)
11. bronchitis	気管支炎 (きかんしえん)
12. pneumonia	肺炎 (はいえん)
13. asthma	喘息 (ぜんそく)
14. tuberculosis (TB)	結核 (けっかく)
15. lung carcinoma[m]; lung cancer	肺がん (はい)
16. gastritis[m]; stomach ache	胃炎 (いえん)
17. food poisoning	食中毒 (しょくちゅうどく)
18. dental caries[m]; cavity	う蝕 (しょく)，虫歯 (むしば)
19. hepatic cirrhosis[m]; cirrhosis of the liver	肝硬変 (かんこうへん)
20. hepatitis	肝炎 (かんえん)
21. stomach ulcer	胃潰瘍 (いかいよう)
22. hemorrhoids; piles	痔核 (じかく)
23. anemia	貧血 (ひんけつ)
24. leukemia	白血病 (はっけつびょう)
25. diabetes mellitus (DM)[m]; diabetes	糖尿病 (とうにょうびょう)

[m] medical word

Part One   Basic medical words

Exercise 1.   Match the English word on the left with a Japanese word on the right.

1. pollinosis   a. 胃炎
2. meningitis   b. 虫歯
3. otitis media   c. 痔核
4. blindness   d. 言語・音声障害
5. bronchitis   e. 視覚障害
6. muteness   f. 髄膜炎
7. gastritis   g. 花粉症
8. hemorrhoids   h. 肝炎
9. hepatitis   i. 中耳炎
10. dental caries   j. 気管支炎

1.____ 2.____ 3.____ 4.____ 5.____ 6.____ 7.____ 8.____ 9.____ 10.____

Exercise 2.   Fill in the missing words or letters to complete these terms. Then write the Japanese in the second space.

日本語

1. laryng_____   _____

2. deaf_____   _____

3. _____ of the liver   _____

4. food_____ing   _____

5. _____ ulcer   _____

6. tuber_____   _____

7. _____ mellitus   _____

8. anem_____   _____

9. _____nia   _____

10. _____ accident   _____

36

Section III   Illnesses and emergencies   Chapter 9

Exercise 3. Complete these sentences with words in the box below. Each word is used only once.

1. Your son has otitis media or a _____. His ear is in pain.

2. You have a large _____. The dentist will fill it next week.

3. I get _____ every spring. My eyes get so itchy!

4. This inhaler will help your daughter breathe when she has an _____ attack.

5. Smoking is one of the common causes of _____.

6. Lin is being treated for _____. Her hair has fallen out.

7. Mrs. Tanaka often gets _____ headaches.

8. It is important to monitor your blood sugar levels when you have _____.

9. Since his _____ my grandfather has had difficulty speaking.

10. It's nothing serious, Mrs. Chen. It's only a _____.

stroke	migraine	anemia	leukemia	lung cancer
middle ear infection		cavity	diabetes	hay fever
asthma		tuberculosis	common cold	

◇ **Dialogue**

Mrs. Ito: My daughter has a high fever and won't stop coughing. She's not drinking any formula and seems to be in terrible pain.

Nurse: Oh my. Can you please take her temperature?

Mrs. Ito: I just did. It's almost 40 degrees. Look, can the doctor see her immediately?

Nurse: The doctor will see her as soon as she can. There are other people waiting now, but you shouldn't have to wait long.

Mrs. Ito: She might have pneumonia. This is an emergency. In my country, patients in serious condition are given priority.

Nurse: I'm sorry, but you'll have to wait your turn. But would you mind taking her temperature? We need to know your daughter's exact condition now so that we can help her.

Part One Basic medical words

Self-study sheet

Write the correct English words in the blanks. Learn them by heart!

1. 脳卒中	
2. 片頭痛	
3. 髄膜炎	
4. 花粉症	
5. 中耳炎	
6. 視覚障害	
7. 聴覚障害	
8. 言語・音声障害	
9. かぜ	
10. 喉頭炎	
11. 気管支炎	
12. 肺炎	
13. 喘息	
14. 結核	
15. 肺がん	
16. 胃炎	
17. 食中毒	
18. 虫歯	
19. 肝硬変	
20. 肝炎	
21. 胃潰瘍	
22. 痔核	
23. 貧血	
24. 白血病	
25. 糖尿病	

You're halfway there! ☺

Section III Illnesses and emergencies

Chapter 10

10. Illnesses and conditions II
Circulatory; Urogenital; Musculoskeletal; Skin; Mental; and Other systems
病気と症状 II — 循環器系，泌尿・生殖器系，筋骨格系，皮膚系，精神系，その他

	Vocabulary	日本語
1.	arteriosclerosis[m]; hardening of the arteries	動脈硬化症 (どうみゃくこうかしょう)
2.	myocardial infarction[m] (MI); heart attack	心筋梗塞，心臓発作 (しんきんこうそく，しんぞうほっさ)
3.	hyperlipidemia[m]; high blood fat	高脂血症 (こうしけっしょう)
4.	hypertension[m]; high blood pressure (HBP)	高血圧 (こうけつあつ)
5.	urinary tract infection (UTI)	尿路感染症 (にょうろかんせんしょう)
6.	renal failure[m]; kidney failure	腎不全 (じんふぜん)
7.	prostatomegaly[m]; enlarged prostate	前立腺肥大症 (ぜんりつせんひだいしょう)
8.	sexually transmitted disease (STD)	性感染症 (せいかんせんしょう)
9.	arthritis	関節炎 (かんせつえん)
10.	rheumatism	リウマチ
11.	gout	痛風 (つうふう)
12.	fungal infection; athlete's foot	水虫，足白癬 (みずむし，そくはくせん)
13.	herpes simplex[m]; cold sore	単純疱疹，口唇ヘルペス（ウイルス性）；疱疹 (たんじゅんほうしん，こうしん／ほうしん)
14.	acne vulgaris[m]; acne	にきび
15.	verruca[m]; wart	いぼ
16.	autism	自閉症 (じへいしょう)
17.	Down syndrome	ダウン症候群 (しょうこうぐん)
18.	clinical depression	うつ病 (びょう)
19.	dementia; senility	認知症 (にんちしょう)
20.	neurosis	神経症 (しんけいしょう)
21.	insomnia	不眠症 (ふみんしょう)
22.	obesity	肥満 (ひまん)
23.	heat stroke; sunstroke	熱中症 (ねっちゅうしょう)
24.	infectious disease	感染症 (かんせんしょう)
25.	chronic illness	慢性疾患 (まんせいしっかん)

[m] medical word

Part One   Basic medical words

Exercise 1.   Match the English word on the left with a Japanese word on the right.

1. arteriosclerosis   a. 不眠症
2. chronic illness   b. 慢性疾患
3. sunstroke   c. うつ病
4. autism   d. 動脈硬化症
5. hyperlipidemia   e. 高脂血症
6. arthritis   f. 熱中症
7. herpes simplex   g. 性感染症
8. sexually transmitted disease   h. 単純疱疹
9. clinical depression   i. 自閉症
10. insomnia   j. 関節炎

1.____ 2.____ 3.____ 4.____ 5.____ 6.____ 7.____ 8.____ 9.____ 10.____

Exercise 2.   Fill in the missing words to complete these terms. Then write the Japanese in the second space.

日本語

1. enlarged _____   _____

2. renal _____   _____

3. Down _____   _____

4. _____ vulgaris   _____

5. _____ sore   _____

6. urinary _____ infection _____

7. myocardial _____   _____

8. hardening of the _____   _____

9. infectious _____   _____

10. _____ foot   _____

40

Section III   Illnesses and emergencies   Chapter 10

Exercise 3. Complete these sentences with words in the box below. Each word is used only once.

1. My grandmother has _____. She can't remember my name.

2. _____ can be controlled through dieting and exercise.

3. You have a _____, and should avoid taking a bath with your child.

4. A sharp pain in your chest may mean you're having a _____.

5. These bumps are _____. The doctor will burn them with liquid nitrogen (液体窒素).

6. _____ refers to problems of the heart, bones, joint, lungs, and kidney.

7. Pimples on the face are symptoms of _____.

8. Obsessive-compulsive disorder (強迫性障害) is a form of _____.

9. Reducing salt in your diet is effective in treating _____.

10. The swelling on your big toe is _____.

hypertension	gout	neurosis	obesity	warts
rheumatism	acne	fungal infection		heat stroke
heart attack		dementia	hyperlipidemia	

◇ Dialogue

Mr. Hodgson is in hospital recovering after surgery for an enlarged prostate.

Nurse: Pardon my directness here, Mr. Hodgson, but how many times did you urinate this morning?

Mr. Hodgson: Twice.

Nurse: Did you experience any pain or discomfort?

Mr. Hodgson: A little, but less than yesterday.

Nurse: Did you notice any blood in the urine this time?

Mr. Hodgson: Yes. It's still a little brownish.

Nurse: Have your bowels moved yet this morning?

Mr. Hodgson: Yes, just after waking up.

Nurse: Were your stools soft or hard?

Mr. Hodgson: Between soft and hard. Just normal, I guess.

Part One   Basic medical words

Self-study sheet

Write the correct English words in the blanks. Learn them by heart!

1. 動脈硬化症	
2. 心臓発作	
3. 高脂血症	
4. 高血圧	
5. 尿路感染症	
6. 腎不全	
7. 前立腺肥大症	
8. 性感染症	
9. 関節炎	
10. リウマチ	
11. 痛風	
12. 水虫	
13. 単純疱疹	
14. にきび	
15. いぼ	
16. 自閉症	
17. ダウン症候群	
18. うつ病	
19. 認知症	
20. 神経症	
21. 不眠症	
22. 肥満	
23. 熱中症	
24. 感染症	
25. 慢性疾患	

Way to go! ☺

11. Children's and women's illnesses and conditions
小児・婦人科の疾患と症状

	Vocabulary	日本語
1.	jaundice	黄疸
2.	sudden infant death syndrome (SIDS)	乳幼児突然死症候群
3.	rubeola ⓜ; measles	麻疹
4.	varicella ⓜ; chickenpox	水痘
5.	parotitis ⓜ; mumps	流行性耳下腺炎
6.	pertussis ⓜ; whooping cough	百日咳
7.	rubella ⓜ; German measles	風疹
8.	acute poliomyelitis ⓜ; polio	急性灰白髄炎，ポリオ
9.	conjunctivitis ⓜ; pink eye	結膜炎
10.	attention deficit hyperactivity disorder ⓜ (ADHD)	注意欠陥多動性障害
11.	candidiasis ⓜ; yeast infection	カンジダ症
12.	cystitis ⓜ	膀胱炎
13.	breast cancer	乳がん
14.	cervical cancer	子宮頚がん
15.	uterine myoma ⓜ; uterine fibroids	子宮筋腫
16.	ovarian cancer	卵巣がん
17.	menopausal disorder	更年期障害
18.	post-partum depression	産後うつ病
19.	amenorrhea ⓜ; absence of periods	無月経
20.	menorrhagia ⓜ; heavy menstrual periods	月経過多
21.	extrauterine pregnancy ⓜ; ectopic pregnancy	子宮外妊娠
22.	nausea and vomiting during pregnancy (NVP) ⓜ; morning sickness	つわり，妊娠悪阻
23.	miscarriage; spontaneous abortion	流産
24.	contractions; labor pains	陣痛
25.	delivery	分娩，出産

ⓜ medical word

Part One   Basic medical words

Exercise 1.   Match the English word on the left with a Japanese word on the right.

1. jaundice   a. 風疹
2. measles   b. 麻疹
3. rubella   c. 急性灰白髄炎
4. breast cancer   d. 子宮頸がん
5. cervical cancer   e. 卵巣がん
6. ovarian cancer   f. 膀胱炎
7. miscarriage   g. 黄疸
8. mumps   h. 乳がん
9. cystitis   i. 流行性耳下腺炎
10. acute poliomyelitis   j. 流産

1.____ 2.____ 3.____ 4.____ 5.____ 6.____ 7.____ 8.____ 9.____ 10.____

Exercise 2.   Fill in the missing words to complete these terms. Then write the Japanese in the second space.

日本語

1. menopausal _____   _____

2. extrauterine _____   _____

3. heavy _____ periods   _____

4. post-_____ depression   _____

5. _____ cough   _____

6. sudden infant death _____ _____

7. yeast _____   _____

8. _____ eye   _____

9. _____ myoma   _____

10. chicken_____   _____

Section III Illnesses and emergencies   Chapter 11

Exercise 3. Complete these sentences with words from the box below. Each word is used only once.

1. Children with _____ may have difficulty paying attention in school.

2. _____ can make the first few months of pregnancy very hard.

3. When your _____ begin, come to the hospital immediately.

4. New parents are often very afraid of _____, though it is rare.

5. Coughing fits are a symptom of _____.

6. Those itchy spots are a sign of _____. But you didn't get it from eating chicken!

7. Will your partner be present at the _____?

8. _____ was first described by German physicians.

9. Women with severe eating disorders may experience an _____.

10. _____ has been called a "silent killer" of women.

delivery	ADHD	mumps	morning sickness	chickenpox
absence of periods		pertussis	German measles	candidiasis
menorrhagia		ovarian cancer	SIDS	contractions

◇ **Dialogue**

Mrs. Cho: Nurse, I'm really worried about my daughter. Jaundice sounds so serious.

Nurse: Don't worry. Jaundice is very common in newborns, especially in Asia. Your daughter just has some excess yellow pigment in her blood.

Mrs. Cho: But the doctor mentioned possible brain damage. My husband and I are worried sick.

Nurse: Only in very rare cases. If your daughter receives phototherapy for a day she should be fine.

Mrs. Cho: But it breaks my heart to see her under those lights. I can't even touch her. Will this treatment cause lasting psychological damage?

Nurse: I promise you it won't. You'll soon be able to hold your daughter. Trust me.

Part One   Basic medical words

Self-study sheet

Write the correct English words in the blanks. Learn them by heart!

1. 黄疸	
2. 乳幼児突然死症候群	
3. 麻疹	
4. 水痘	
5. 流行性耳下腺炎	
6. 百日咳	
7. 風疹	
8. 急性灰白髄炎	
9. 結膜炎	
10. 注意欠陥多動性障害	
11. カンジダ症	
12. 膀胱炎	
13. 乳がん	
14. 子宮頸がん	
15. 子宮筋腫	
16. 卵巣がん	
17. 更年期障害	
18. 産後うつ病	
19. 無月経	
20. 月経過多	
21. 子宮外妊娠	
22. つわり	
23. 流産	
24. 陣痛	
25. 分娩	

It's all downhill from here! 🙂

Section III Illnesses and emergencies

Chapter 12

12. Injuries and emergencies
外傷と救急

Vocabulary (n)	日本語	Variations (n & v)
1. cramp	こむら返り	Her leg muscles **cramped** while swimming.
2. sprain	捻挫	You've **sprained** your ankle.
3. dislocation	脱臼	You've **dislocated** your shoulder.
4. fracture; broken bone	骨折	You've **fractured** your wrist. Your wrist is **broken**.
5. wound; cut	創傷, 傷	Her arm was **wounded** in the crash.
6. injury	けが	He has been **injured** many times.
7. scrape	擦過傷	He fell and **scraped** his knee.
8. laceration	裂傷	Her leg was **lacerated** in the accident.
9. burn	熱傷	He **burned** his hand while cooking.
10. blister	水疱	She has painful **blisters** on her feet.
11. bruise	打撲傷	He has a **bruise** under his eye.
12. scar	傷跡	I am afraid this will leave a **scar**.
13. lump	腫瘤, しこり	She found a **lump** in her breast.
14. to choke (on something) (v)	(何かを)のどに詰まらせる	The boy was **choking** on some bread.
15. asphyxiation⑩; suffocation	窒息	The girl nearly **suffocated** in the car.
16. to attempt suicide (v)	自殺を図る	She **attempted suicide** by swallowing sleeping pills.
17. to drown (v)	溺水する	He nearly **drowned** in the river.
18. hypothermia	低体温	He has **hypothermia**.
19. seizure	痙攣	Hurry! She's having a **seizure**!
20. paralysis	麻痺	Your father is **paralyzed**.
21. concussion	脳しんとう	He has a **concussion**.
22. coma, comatose (adj)	昏睡状態	He is now in a **coma**.
23. unconscious	意識不明	He is **unconscious**. He **lost consciousness** two hours ago.
24. artificial respiration	人工呼吸	He is on **artificial respiration**.
25. cardiopulmonary resuscitation⑩ (CPR)	心肺蘇生法	They administered **CPR** but could not revive him.

⑩ medical word

Part One Basic medical words

Exercise 1. Match the English word on the left with a Japanese word on the right.

1. dislocation
2. injury
3. burn
4. to choke
5. suffocation
6. hypothermia
7. paralysis
8. bruise
9. unconscious
10. fracture

a. 窒息
b. 骨折
c. 脱臼
d. 意識不明
e. けが
f. 低体温
g. 熱傷
h. 麻痺
i. のどに詰まらせる
j. 打撲傷

1.____ 2.____ 3.____ 4.____ 5.____ 6.____ 7.____ 8.____ 9.____ 10.____

Exercise 2. Put these words in the correct order. Write the sentence on the line.

1. her cramped muscles swimming while leg   _____

2. seizure is she a having   _____

3. knee fell his and he scraped   _____

4. ago he lost two hours consciousness   _____

5. found in her she breast lump a   _____

6. drowned he in nearly river the   _____

7. your paralyzed father is   _____

8. concussion he a has   _____

9. sprained your you have ankle   _____

10. is broken wrist your   _____

48

Section III Illnesses and emergencies   Chapter 12

Exercise 3. Fill in the blanks with the missing verbs (動詞) or prepositions (前置詞).

1. Her arm _____ badly wounded in the traffic accident.

2. I _____ painful blisters on my feet.

3. Don't be alarmed, but I have _____ a tiny lump in your breast.

4. I'm afraid that this cut will _____ a scar.

5. Your grandmother is _____ a coma now.

6. The EMTs _____ CPR but could not revive the man.

7. Edgar has been _____ artificial respiration for three days.

8. Xian _____ suicide by mixing dangerous chemicals.

9. Her forearms _____ lacerated by a man with a knife.

10. Your mother has _____ consciousness again.

lost	were	have	leave	to
on	administered	gave	in	attempted
did	found	was	by	

◇ Dialogue

Mr. Pimiento has come to the emergency ward after falling from his bicycle.

Nurse: Your knee is badly scraped, Mr. Pimiento, but you're lucky you weren't injured more seriously.

Mr. Pimiento: I know. I guess I'm not used to riding a bicycle in Japan.

Nurse: All right, I have to disinfect your scrape and clean out the gravel and dirt.

Mr. Pimiento: Oh. That sounds painful.

Nurse: It will sting a bit, but it should be over soon. Could you please extend your leg? Please let me know if the pain becomes severe.

(The nurse cleans out the scrape.)

Nurse: There! You're all set. That wasn't so bad, was it?

Mr. Pimiento: Well, you were right, it did sting a little. Will this leave a scar?

Nurse: I don't think so. It should heal nicely.

Part One   Basic medical words

Self-study sheet

Write the correct English words in the blanks. Learn them by heart!

1. こむら返り	
2. 捻挫	
3. 脱臼	
4. 骨折	
5. 創傷	
6. けが	
7. 擦過傷	
8. 裂傷	
9. 熱傷	
10. 水疱	
11. 打撲傷	
12. 傷跡	
13. しこり	
14. のどに詰まらせる	
15. 窒息	
16. 自殺を図る	
17. 溺水する	
18. 低体温	
19. 痙攣	
20. 麻痺	
21. 脳しんとう	
22. 昏睡状態	
23. 意識不明	
24. 人工呼吸	
25. 心肺蘇生法	

Marvelous! ☺

Part Two
Basic communication
基本的なコミュニケーション表現

Section IV   Nurse-to-patient communication　患者とのコミュニケーション

- Chapter **13**　Common complaints　主訴
- Chapter **14**　Taking a patient's history　病歴の聴取
- Chapter **15**　Giving instructions during an examination　検査時の助言
- Chapter **16**　Common questions from foreign patients　外国人患者がよく問う質問

Section V   Communication and encouragement　コミュニケーションと励ましの言葉

- Chapter **17**　Daily routine communication　看護師の日常会話
- Chapter **18**　Words of encouragement　励ましの言葉

Section IV　Nurse-to-patient communication

Chapter 13

13. Common complaints
主訴

Sentences	日本語
1. I feel feverish (hot).	体が熱っぽい（熱い）です．
2. My eyes are itchy.	目がかゆいです．
3. When I stand up I feel dizzy.	立ちくらみがします．
4. I have a splitting (pounding) headache.	頭が割れそうに（ずきずき）痛みます．
5. I can't stand this earache.	耳が痛くて耐えられません．
6. I have sneezing fits all day.	一日中，くしゃみが出ます．
7. I have a runny nose. (My nose is running.)	鼻水が出ます．
8. My nose is all stuffed up.	鼻が詰まっています．
9. I feel short of breath. ☺	息切れがします．
10. It hurts when I breathe.	息をすると胸が痛みます．
11. Sometimes my heart races.	ときどき脈が速くなります．
12. My throat is sore.	喉が痛いです．
13. I have a dry cough.	かわいた咳が出ます．
14. I have a productive cough. (I've been coughing up phlegm.)	咳が痰を伴います． 咳をすると痰が出ます．
15. I feel nauseous.	吐き気がします．
16. I vomited twice this morning.	今朝，2回吐きました．
17. I have diarrhea (the runs).	下痢をしています．
18. I'm constipated.	便秘をしています．
19. I perspire (sweat) a lot at night.	寝汗がひどいです．
20. I can't sleep at night.	夜眠れません．
21. I feel fatigue (tired, sluggish, dull).	体がだるいです．
22. I'm always thirsty.	いつも喉が渇いています．
23. My period is four weeks late.	生理が4週間遅れています．
24. I'm worried about this rash.	この発疹が気になっています．
25. I haven't been myself lately.	最近調子が悪いです．

☺ shortness of breath = dyspnea; The patient is *dyspneic* ⓜ.
ⓜ medical word

Part Two   Basic communication

Exercise 1.   Match the English expression on the left with a Japanese expression on the right.

1. I'm worried about this rash.
2. When I stand up I feel dizzy.
3. I can't stand this earache.
4. I can't sleep at night.
5. My period is late.
6. My throat is sore.
7. I feel nauseous.
8. I have diarrhea
9. I feel short of breath.
10. I'm always thirsty.

a. 耳が痛くて耐えられません．
b. この発疹が気になっています．
c. 息切れがします．
d. 生理が遅れています．
e. 吐き気がします．
f. 喉が痛いです．
g. いつも喉が渇いています．
i. 立ちくらみがします．
j. 夜眠れません．
k. 下痢をしています．

1.____ 2.____ 3.____ 4.____ 5.____ 6.____ 7.____ 8.____ 9.____ 10.____

Exercise 2.   Read the following sentences and <u>underline</u> the correct word in parentheses ( ). Then rewrite the complete sentence on the line.

1. My heart is (racing / sluggish). _____

2. I'm (worry / worried) about this rash. _____

3. I (sweet / sweat) a lot at night. _____

4. It (aches / hurts) when I breathe. _____

5. I have (sneezing / vomiting) fits all day. _____

6. I have a dry (cough / nose). _____

7. My nose is all (stuffy / stuffed up). _____

8. I have a (splitting / racing) headache. _____

9. I haven't been (me / myself) lately. _____

10. I feel so (tiring / sluggish). _____

54

Exercise 3. Complete these sentences with words in the box below.

N. What seems to be the problem?

P. It (1)_____ when I breathe and I've been coughing up (2)_____.

N. Do you have any other symptoms?

P. Yes. I (3)_____ twice this morning.

N. Do you feel (4)_____?

P. Yes, I'm hot, and I'm (5)_____, too. My bowels haven't moved for three days.

N. What seems to be the trouble?

P. I have a (6)_____ nose and I've had (7)_____ fits all day. And I have a (8)_____ throat.

N. Hmm. You're running a low-grade fever, too. Anything else?

P. My eyes are (9)_____ and I have a (10)_____ headache. It's like someone is hitting my head with a hammer. I'm just in bad shape!

itchy	thirsty	phlegm	pounding	sore
runny	sneezing	feverish		fatigue
vomited	hurts	constipated	splitting	

◇ Dialogue

Nurse: Since you're a first-time patient you need to fill in this form. Could you write your name, address, phone number and date of birth here? Romaji is fine.

(After Miss Wei fills in the form)

Nurse: And what brings you here today?

Miss Wei: Well, I have this persistent cough. I can't stop coughing! My nose is running, too.

Nurse: Have you noticed any coloration in the nasal drainage (鼻水)?

Miss Wei: Yes, it's kind of yellowish. Does this mean I have an infection?

Nurse: The doctor will be able to answer that question. Please have a seat and wait until your name is called.

Part Two   Basic communication

Self-study sheet

Write the correct English sentences in the blanks. Learn them by heart!

1. 体が熱っぽいです．	
2. 目がかゆいです．	
3. 立ちくらみがします．	
4. 頭が割れそうに痛みます．	
5. 耳が痛くて耐えられません．	
6. 一日中，くしゃみが出ます．	
7. 鼻水が出ます．	
8. 鼻が詰まっています．	
9. 息切れがします．	
10. 息をすると胸が痛みます．	
11. ときどき脈が速くなります．	
12. 喉が痛いです．	
13. かわいた咳が出ます．	
14. 咳をすると痰が出ます．	
15. 吐き気がします．	
16. 今朝，２回吐きました．	
17. 下痢をしています．	
18. 便秘をしています．	
19. 寝汗がひどいです．	
20. 夜眠れません．	
21. 体がだるいです．	
22. いつも喉が渇いています．	
23. 生理が４週間遅れています．	
24. この発疹が気になっています．	
25. 最近調子が悪いです．	

Well done! ☺

Section IV　Nurse-to-patient communication

14. Taking a patient's history
病歴の聴取

Sentences	日本語
1. Do you smoke?	タバコを吸いますか.
2. How many cigarettes (packs) do you smoke per day?	1日に何本（何箱）くらいタバコを吸いますか.
3. How is your appetite?	食欲はありますか.
4. Do you have regular bowel movements?	規則正しい便通がありますか.
5. How many times do you urinate in a day?	排尿は1日に何回ありますか.
6. Are your periods regular?	月経は規則正しくありますか.
7. When was your last period?	最終月経はいつでしたか.
8. Are you sleeping well?	よく眠れますか.
9. What is your occupation (job)?	ご職業は何ですか.
10. Do you have a lot of stress in your work?	お仕事ではストレスが多いですか.
11. Do you exercise regularly?	定期的に運動しますか.
12. Are you married?	ご結婚されていますか.
13. Has anyone in your family been hospitalized for a serious illness?	ご家族の中に大きな病気で入院された方はいらっしゃいますか.
14. Is there a history of heart problems in your family?	ご家族の中で心臓病にかかったことがある方はいらっしゃいますか.
15. Have you ever had a serious illness before?	これまでに大きな病気をしたことがありますか.
16. Do you have any chronic illnesses?	慢性の病気はありますか.
17. Do you have any allergies?	何かアレルギーはありますか.
18. Are you allergic to any medications?	薬に対するアレルギーはありますか.
19. Are you taking any medication (supplements) now?	何か薬（サプリメント）を飲んでいますか.
20. How long have you had this fever?	熱はどのくらい続いていますか.

Part Two   Basic communication

Exercise 1.   Match the English expression on the left with a Japanese expression on the right.

1. How many packs do you smoke per day?
2. Are you married?
3. How is your appetite?
4. When was your last period?
5. Are you allergic to any medications?
6. Has anyone in your family been hospitalized for a serious illness?
7. Is there a history of heart problems in your family?
8. Are you taking any supplements now?
9. Do you have a lot of stress in your work?
10. Do you have regular bowel movements?

a. 最終月経はいつでしたか．
b. １日に何箱くらいタバコを吸いますか．
c. 食欲はありますか．
d. ご結婚されていますか．
e. ご家族の中に大きな病気で入院された方はいらっしゃいますか．
f. 何かサプリメントを飲んでいますか．
g. お仕事ではストレスが多いですか．
h. ご家族の中に心臓病にかかったことがある方はいらっしゃいますか．
i. 薬に対するアレルギーはありますか．
j. 規則正しい便通がありますか．

1.____ 2.____ 3.____ 4.____ 5.____ 6.____ 7.____ 8.____ 9.____ 10.____

Exercise 2.   Make sentences by connecting these phrases. Rewrite each complete sentence below.

1. Are you allergic
2. How long have you had
3. Do you
4. Do you have
5. Has anyone in your family
6. How many times do you
7. Have you ever had
8. Are you
9. What is
10. Are your

a. periods regular?
b. any chronic illnesses?
c. this fever?
d. sleeping well?
e. your occupation?
f. to any medications?
g. a serious illness before?
h. been hospitalized for a serious illness?
i. exercise regularly?
j. urinate in a day?

1. _____
2. _____
3. _____
4. _____
5. _____
6. _____
7. _____
8. _____
9. _____
10. _____

Exercise 3. Read the patient's answers and fill in the nurse's questions.

N. (1)_____?
P. Chronic? Well, I had asthma when I was a child, but now I'm fine.

N. (2)_____?
P. Yes, I had pneumonia two or three times as a child. Nothing more serious than that, though.

N. (3)_____?
P. Yes, my father and grandfather both had heart problems.

N. (4)_____?
P. Yes. I do. I smoke a pack a day.

N. (5)_____?
P. Just fine. In fact I'm hungry now.

N. (6)_____?
P. Not regularly, but I sometimes cycle to work.

N. (7)_____?
P. Yes, I'm allergic to house dust and mold.

N. (8)_____?
P. Yes, I take some medicine to control my allergies.

N. (9)_____?
P. Yes, they are. Every 29 days.

N. (10)_____?
P. Last week.

◇ Dialogue

Mr. McDermott is having a yearly health check-up.

Nurse:	I hope you don't mind, but I have to ask a few questions about your lifestyle.
Mr. McDermott:	Sure, go right ahead.
Nurse:	First of all, do you smoke?
Mr. McDermott:	Nope. Never smoked in my life.
Nurse:	Do you drink alcohol?
Mr. McDermott:	Yes, that I do.
Nurse:	How much alcohol do you drink in a day?
Mr. McDermott:	Not every day. On weekends, mostly.
Nurse:	What kind of drink, and how much?
Mr. McDermott:	Beer, usually. One or two cans each time.

Part Two Basic communication

Self-study sheet

Write the correct English sentences in the blanks. Learn them by heart!

1. タバコを吸いますか.	
2. １日に何本くらいタバコを吸いますか.	
3. 食欲はありますか.	
4. 規則正しい便通がありますか.	
5. 排尿は１日に何回ありますか.	
6. 月経は規則正しくありますか.	
7. 最終月経はいつでしたか.	
8. よく眠れますか.	
9. ご職業は何ですか.	
10. お仕事ではストレスが多いですか.	
11. 定期的に運動しますか.	
12. ご結婚されていますか.	
13. ご家族の中に大きな病気で入院された方はいらっしゃいますか.	
14. ご家族の中で心臓病にかかったことがある方はいらっしゃいますか.	
15. これまでに大きな病気をしたことがありますか.	
16. 慢性の病気はありますか.	
17. 何かアレルギーはありますか.	
18. 薬に対するアレルギーはありますか.	
19. 何か薬を飲んでいますか.	
20. 熱はどのくらい続いていますか.	

You've made great progress! ☺

Section IV Nurse-to-patient communication

Chapter 15

15. Giving instructions during an examination
検査時の助言

	Sentences	日本語
1.	Please wait in front of the examination room.	検査室の前でお待ちください．
2.	Please keep this thermometer under your arm until it beeps.	ピーと鳴るまで体温計を腋の下にはさんでおいてください．
3.	I'm going to take your blood pressure.	血圧を測ります．
4.	Please roll up your sleeve.	袖をまくってください．
5.	I'm going to take a blood sample.	採血します．
6.	Please give me your right arm.	右手を出してください．
7.	Now make a fist.	握りこぶしを作ってください．
8.	This may prick a little.	チクッとしますよ．
9.	Hold still for a moment.	しばらく動かないでください．
10.	Next you need to give a urine sample.	次は尿検査です．
11.	Please fill this cup about one-third full.	カップの1/3まで尿を入れてください．
12.	We're going to take a chest X-ray.	胸の写真をとります．
13.	Please take off your shirt.	上着を脱いでください．
14.	You can leave on your t-shirt (bra).	T-シャツ（ブラジャー）を着たままでいいですよ．
15.	Take a deep breath and hold it.	息を深く吸って，止めてください．
16.	Breathe in and out slowly.	ゆっくり息を吸ったり吐いたりしてください．
17.	Please lie down on the bed.	ベッドに横になってください．
18.	Please roll over onto your stomach.	うつ伏せになってください．
19.	You can sit up now.	どうぞ起き上がってください．
20.	Go ahead and relax.	力をぬいてください．

Part Two　Basic communication

Exercise 1.　Match the English expression on the left with a Japanese expression on the right.

1. Please wait in front of the examination room.
2. I'm going to take your blood pressure.
3. You can leave on your bra.
4. Now make a fist.
5. Go ahead and relax.
6. Please roll over onto your stomach.
7. We're going to take a chest X-ray.
8. Please lie down on the bed.
9. Take a deep breath and hold it.
10. Next you need to give a urine sample.

a. 次は尿検査です．
b. 検査室の前でお待ちください．
c. 血圧を測ります．
d. 握りこぶしを作ってください．
e. 息を深く吸って，止めてください．
f. ブラジャーを着たままでいいですよ．
g. 胸の写真をとります．
h. うつ伏せになってください．
i. 力をぬいてください．
j. ベッドに横になってください．

1.___　2.___　3.___　4.___　5.___　6.___　7.___　8.___　9.___　10.___

Exercise 2.　Make sentences by connecting these phrases. Rewrite each complete sentence below.

1. I'm going to take
2. Please roll up
3. Please give me
4. This may
5. Please fill this cup
6. Please take off
7. Breathe in
8. Please lie down
9. Please roll over
10. You can

a. your sleeve.
b. prick a little.
c. onto your stomach.
d. and out slowly.
e. on the bed.
f. a blood sample.
g. about one-third full.
h. your shirt.
i. sit up now.
j. your right arm.

1. _____
2. _____
3. _____
4. _____
5. _____
6. _____
7. _____
8. _____
9. _____
10. _____

Section IV Nurse-to-patient communication   Chapter 15

Exercise 3. Read the answers and fill in the nurse's lines. This is *not* one long conversation.

N. (1)_____
P. Blood sample? All right, but I really hate needles.

N. (2)_____
P. About one-third, OK. Where should I put this cup when I finish?

N. (3)_____
P. OK. Is it rolled up far enough?

N. (4)_____
P. All right. Will I have to wait long for the doctor?

N. (5)_____
P. Should I take off my shoes before lying down?

N. (6)_____
P. I'd prefer my left, actually.

N. (7)_____
P. I really don't like X-rays.

N. (8)_____
P. (*Pause*). I don't think this is working. I didn't hear any beep.

N. (9)_____
P. I am holding still.

N. (10)_____
P. Do I have to take off my t-shirt, too?

◇ **Dialogue**

Nurse: I'll check your height and weight. Please take off your shoes and step on this scale.
Mr. Thomas: All right.
Nurse: 71.5 kilograms. Now let's measure your height. Step on this scale here. Keep your back straight. Good. 165 cm. Please have a seat here and wait until your name is called.

(*A few minutes passes*).

Nurse: Mr. Thomas, please come in. Have a seat here. Which arm would you prefer?
Mr. Thomas: Oh, my right one.
Nurse: Please roll up your sleeve. Relax. You'll just feel a pinch. There, all finished. Hold this cotton swab here for a moment. Good. Please return to the waiting room. You'll have to wait 20 minutes before leaving.

Part Two　Basic communication

Self-study sheet

Write the correct English sentences in the blanks.　Learn them by heart!

1.　検査室の前でお待ちください．	
2.　ピーと鳴るまで体温計を腋の下にはさんでおいてください．	
3.　血圧を測ります．	
4.　袖をまくってください．	
5.　採血します．	
6.　右手を出してください．	
7.　握りこぶしを作ってください．	
8.　チクッとしますよ．	
9.　しばらく動かないでください．	
10.　次は尿検査です．	
11.　カップの1/3まで尿を入れてください．	
12.　胸の写真をとります．	
13.　上着を脱いでください．	
14.　T-シャツを着たままでいいですよ．	
15.　息を深く吸って，止めてください．	
16.　ゆっくり息を吸ったり吐いたりしてください．	
17.　ベッドに横になってください．	
18.　うつ伏せになってください．	
19.　どうぞ起き上がってください．	
20.　力をぬいてください．	

Nicely done! ☺

16. Common questions from foreign patients
外国人患者がよく問う質問

	Sentences	日本語
1.	What does this medicine do?	この薬は何のためですか.
2.	Does this medicine have any side effects?	この薬に何か副作用はありますか.
3.	This medicine isn't working. Can you change it?	この薬は効きません. 変えてもらえませんか.
4.	How long will this IV take?	点滴はどのくらい時間がかかりますか.
5.	What do I need to bring with me when I'm hospitalized?	入院するときに必要な持ち物は何ですか.
6.	How many days do I have to be hospitalized?	入院は何日間ぐらいですか.
7.	Where should I keep my valuables (clothes)?	貴重品（衣服）はどこに置けばいいですか.
8.	Can I see the doctor now?	今主治医に会えますか.
9.	Does this meal contain pork (meat)?	この食事には豚肉（肉）が入っていますか.
10.	Is the X-ray machine safe?	X線は安全ですか.
11.	When will the test results be ready?	検査の結果はいつわかりますか.
12.	Is it OK if I eat before the operation?	手術の前に食べてもいいですか.
13.	I'm really nervous. Could you please stay with me?	緊張しています. 私のそばにいてくれませんか.
14.	Will the operation (test) be painful?	手術（検査）は痛みますか.
15.	Will I be awake during the operation?	手術中は目が覚めていますか.
16.	How did the operation go?	手術はうまくいきましたか.
17.	Can I be transferred to a private room?	個室に移ることはできますか.
18.	Can I take a shower now?	今シャワーを浴びてもいいですか.
19.	I'm feeling better. Can I check out early?	だいぶ良くなりました. 早く退院してもいいですか.
20.	Can you explain the check out procedures?	退院の手続きを教えてもらえませんか.

Part Two   Basic communication

Exercise 1.   Match the English expression on the left with a Japanese expression on the right.

1. Can you explain the check out procedures?
2. Can I take a shower now?
3. Will the operation be painful?
4. Is it OK if I eat before the operation?
5. Can I see the doctor now?
6. How long will this IV take?
7. Does this medicine have any side effects?
8. What does this medicine do?
9. Does this meal contain meat?
10. What do I need to bring with me when I'm hospitalized?

a. 今シャワーを浴びてもいいですか．
b. 手術の前に食べてもいいですか．
c. 今主治医に会えますか．
d. この薬に何か副作用はありますか．
e. 退院の手続きを教えてもらえませんか．
f. 入院するときに必要な持ち物は何ですか．
g. 点滴はどのくらい時間がかかりますか．
h. この食事には肉が入っていますか．
i. この薬は何のためですか．
j. 手術は痛みますか．

1.____ 2.____ 3.____ 4.____ 5.____ 6.____ 7.____ 8.____ 9.____ 10.____

Exercise 2.   Fill in the question word. Then rewrite each question below.

1. _____ the X-ray machine safe?
2. _____ many days do I have to be hospitalized?
3. _____ this medicine have any side effects?
4. _____ should I keep my valuables?
5. _____ this meal contain pork?
6. _____ will the test results be ready?
7. _____ you please stay with me?
8. _____ the operation be painful?
9. _____ does this medicine do?
10. _____ long will this IV take?

1. _____
2. _____
3. _____
4. _____
5. _____
6. _____
7. _____
8. _____
9. _____
10. _____

Section IV Nurse-to-patient communication   Chapter 16

Exercise 3. Read the answers and fill in the patient's questions. This is *not* one long conversation.

P. (1)_____
N. I'm sorry but it is still too soon for you to check out.

P. (2)_____
N. No, you will be asleep during the operation.

P. (3)_____
N. They'll be ready in about an hour.

P. (4)_____
N. You will need to be here for about two or three days.

P. (5)_____
N. Pajamas, a towel, underwear, eating utensils and toiletries.

P. (6)_____
N. It went very well.

P. (7)_____
N. I'm sorry, none are available now.

P. (8)_____
N. The doctor is doing his rounds now but will be back in the afternoon.

P. (9)_____
N. It may take a little time for the medicine to work. Please be patient.

P. (10)_____
N. No, you shouldn't eat anything on the day of the operation.

◇ Dialogue

Patient: I've never seen medicine like this before. How do I take it?
Nurse: This is powdered medicine. Just open the bag and swallow it, and wash it down with a glass of water.
Patient: I see. But there's only a three day prescription. Can't I get a one week supply?
Nurse: I'm afraid not. The doctor wrote only a three day prescription.
Patient: But what if I'm still sick after three days? I'll need more medicine.
Nurse: If the medicine is not effective after three days you can come back in for a different prescription. How about that?
Patient: Well, OK. Oh, the doctor also said I was "febrile." That sounds scary. What does it mean?
Nurse: It just means you have a fever. I apologize if we caused you any alarm.

Part Two　Basic communication

Self-study sheet

Write the correct English sentences in the blanks. Learn them by heart!

1.　この薬は何のためですか．	
2.　この薬に何か副作用はありますか．	
3.　この薬は効きません．変えてもらえませんか．	
4.　点滴はどのくらい時間がかかりますか．	
5.　入院するときに必要な持ち物は何ですか．	
6.　入院は何日間ぐらいですか．	
7.　貴重品はどこに置けばいいですか．	
8.　今主治医に会えますか．	
9.　この食事には豚肉が入っていますか．	
10.　X線は安全ですか．	
11.　検査の結果はいつわかりますか．	
12.　手術の前に食べてもいいですか．	
13.　緊張しています．私のそばにいてくれませんか．	
14.　手術は痛みますか．	
15.　手術中は目が覚めていますか．	
16.　手術はうまくいきましたか．	
17.　個室に移ることはできますか．	
18.　今シャワーを浴びてもいいですか．	
19.　だいぶ良くなりました．早く退院してもいいですか．	
20.　退院の手続きを教えてもらえませんか．	

Just a little more to go! ☺

Section V　Communication and encouragement

Chapter 17

17. Daily routine communication
看護師の日常会話

Sentences	日本語
1. Excuse me. May I come in?	失礼します．
2. I'm Ken Kagawa. I'll be your primary nurse.	担当看護師のケン・カガワです．
3. I can speak a little English.	私は少し英語を話せます．
4. Are you familiar with procedures in a Japanese hospital (clinic)?	日本の病院（医院）の手続きなどはおわかりですか．
5. Do you have a health insurance card?	保険証はお持ちですか．
6. Do you have any questions (concerns)?	何かご質問（心配事）はありますか．
7. Please do not use your cellular phone in this room.	この部屋では携帯電話を使わないでください．
8. Press the call button if you need anything.	もし何かあればナースコールを押してください．
9. Are there any foods that you cannot eat?	食べられないものはありますか．
10. Please return your tray to the cart after you've finished.	食べ終わったらトレイをカートにお返しください．
11. How was your meal?	食事はどうでしたか．
12. You may take a bath from 8:00 am to 8:00 pm.	お風呂は午前8:00から午後8:00まで入れます．
13. You need your own towel and toiletries.	タオルや洗面用具はご自分でご用意ください．
14. Did you take your medicine?	薬は飲まれましたか．
15. Please let me know if you feel any pain (discomfort).	痛み（不快な感じ）があれば言ってください．
16. Could you please speak more slowly?	もう少しゆっくり話してください．
17. Pardon me? (Could you repeat that?)	もう一度言ってください．
18. I'm sorry to disturb your rest.	お休み中すみません．
19. Sorry to have kept you waiting.	お待たせしました．
20. Visiting hours are over. You'll have to go now.	面会時間は終わりました．お帰りください．

Part Two　Basic communication

Exercise 1.　Match the English expression on the left with a Japanese expression on the right.

1. Excuse me. May I come in?
2. I can speak a little English.
3. Do you have a health insurance card?
4. Press the call button if you need anything.
5. You may take a bath from 8:00 am to 8:00 pm.
6. Did you take your medicine?
7. Could you please speak more slowly?
8. Could you repeat that?
9. Sorry to have kept you waiting.
10. Do you have any questions?

a. 保険証はお持ちですか．
b. 薬は飲まれましたか．
c. もう一度言ってください．
d. お待たせしました．
e. もし何かあればナースコールを押してください．
f. 何かご質問はありますか．
g. 失礼します．
h. 私は少し英語を話せます．
i. もう少しゆっくり話してください．
j. お風呂は午前 8:00 から午後 8:00 まで入れます．

1.___　2.___　3.___　4.___　5.___　6.___　7.___　8.___　9.___　10.___

Exercise 2.　Put these words in the correct order. Write the sentence on the line.

1. primary I'll your nurse be　_____
2. disturb sorry rest your I'm to　_____
3. toiletries your towel need you own and　_____
4. pain know please let you if me feel any　_____
5. waiting to sorry kept you have I'm　_____
6. was your meal how　_____
7. are visiting over hours　_____
8. need you if press anything call the button　_____
9. you could please more speak slowly　_____
10. card you have do insurance health a　_____

Section V Communication and encouragement   Chapter 17

Exercise 3. Read the answers and fill in the nurse's or patient's line. This is *not* one long conversation.

N. (1)_____

P. Sure, come in.

N. (2)_____

P. Well, where can I use it then?

N. (3)_____

P. Oops, I forgot. I'll take it now.

N. (4)_____

P. Not right now. You've explained everything very well.

N. (5)_____

P. Yes, I think so. This is my third time to stay in a Japanese hospital.

P. I'm worried about the food here.

N. Hmm. (6)_____

P. What should I do with this tray when I'm done eating?

N. (7)_____

P. I feel really grubby. When can I take a bath?

N. (8)_____

P. Nurse, I have a question about (*mumble*).

N. (9)_____

P. I can't speak Japanese. Does anyone on staff speak English?

N. (10)_____

◇ **Dialogue**

Nurse:	It's time to take your temperature again, Mr. Owuru. How was your lunch?
Mr. Owuru:	Oh, it was not so bad. Better than breakfast.
Nurse:	How much of your lunch were you able to eat?
Mr. Owuru:	All of it. Actually, I'm still hungry.
Nurse:	Your appetite seems to be fine. But oh, you're still running a fever.
Mr. Owuru:	I'm feeling better, though. I would like to take a walk outside of the hospital, in fact. Some fresh air would do me good.
Nurse:	I can ask the doctor about that, but I think you need more rest. How about a walk around the hospital?
Mr. Owuru:	All right. I guess I can wait one more day.

Part Two　Basic communication

Self-study sheet

Write the correct English sentences in the blanks. Learn them by heart!

1. 失礼します.	
2. 担当看護師のケン・カガワです.	
3. 私は少し英語を話せます.	
4. 日本の病院の手続きなどはおわかりですか.	
5. 保険証はお持ちですか.	
6. 何かご質問はありますか.	
7. この部屋では携帯電話を使わないでください.	
8. もし何かあればナースコールを押してください.	
9. 食べられないものはありますか.	
10. 食べ終わったらトレイをカートにお返しください.	
11. 食事はどうでしたか.	
12. お風呂は午前 8:00 から午後 8:00 まで入れます.	
13. タオルや洗面用具はご自分でご用意ください.	
14. 薬は飲まれましたか.	
15. 痛みがあれば言ってください.	
16. もう少しゆっくり話してください.	
17. もう一度言ってください.	
18. お休み中すみません.	
19. お待たせしました.	
20. 面会時間は終わりました. お帰りください.	

Fantastic! ☺

Section V　Communication and encouragement

Chapter 18

18. Words of encouragement
励ましの言葉

	Sentences	日本語
1.	How are you feeling?	ご気分はいかがですか．
2.	Can I get you anything?	何か持ってきましょうか．
3.	Don't worry. Everything will be fine.	心配しないで．大丈夫ですよ．
4.	There's no need to panic.	慌てないでください．
5.	Here, let me help you.	お手伝いしましょうか．
6.	I understand. (I see.)	わかりました．
7.	You're doing great.	順調ですよ．
8.	I'm sure you can do it.	きっとできますよ．
9.	Let's give it another try.	もう一度やってみましょう．
10.	Keep going.	続けてください．
11.	That's perfect!	完璧です．
12.	Shall we take a break?	少し休みましょうか．
13.	You look a bit pale.	ちょっと顔色が悪いですね．
14.	Do you need to lie down?	横になりたいのですか．
15.	I'll stay with you for a while.	しばらくおそばにいますよ．
16.	This must be very difficult for you.	おつらいですね．
17.	I hope you feel better soon.	早く元気になるといいですね．
18.	The worst is behind you.	一番大変なところはもう終わりました．
19.	You need to get some rest.	安静が必要ですよ．
20.	Please take care of yourself.	お大事になさってください．

73

Part Two   Basic communication

Exercise 1.   Match the English expression on the left with a Japanese expression on the right.

1. How are you feeling?
2. Don't worry. Everything will be fine.
3. Here, let me help you.
4. I'm sure you can do it.
5. That's perfect!
6. Keep going.
7. I'll stay with you for a while.
8. I hope you feel better soon.
9. Please take care of yourself.
10. Do you need to lie down?

a. お大事になさってください．
b. ご気分はいかがですか．
c. 完璧です．
d. しばらくおそばにいますよ．
e. 早く元気になるといいですね．
f. 心配しないで．大丈夫ですよ．
g. お手伝いしましょうか．
h. 横になりたいのですか．
i. 続けてください．
j. きっとできますよ．

1.____   2.____   3.____   4.____   5.____   6.____   7.____   8.____   9.____   10.____

Exercise 2.   Make sentences by connecting these phrases. Rewrite each complete sentence below.

1. Can I get
2. There's no need
3. I'm sure
4. Shall we
5. You're doing
6. You need
7. Let's give it
8. You look
9. The worst is
10. This must be

a. to panic.
b. very difficult for you.
c. a bit pale.
d. you anything?
e. another try.
f. you can do it.
g. take a break?
h. great.
i. to get some rest.
j. behind you.

1. _____
2. _____
3. _____
4. _____
5. _____
6. _____
7. _____
8. _____
9. _____
10. _____

Section V   Communication and encouragement   Chapter 18

Exercise 3. Read the answers and fill in the nurse's or patient's line. This is *not* one long conversation.

N. (1)_____

P. I'm feeling much better, thanks.

N. (2)_____

P. Thanks for staying. I appreciate your company.

N. (3)_____

P. Pale? Well, I feel like I might vomit.

N. (4)_____

P. Good idea. I could use a break.

N. (5)_____

P. O.K. I'll give it another shot.

P. I think I need some help getting out of bed.

N. (6)_____

P. My son is allergic to dairy products.

N. (7)_____. He'll have special non-dairy meals.

P. I'm a little worried about the operation tomorrow.

N. (8)_____

P. Today's therapy was really hard. Will it be as hard tomorrow?

N. I don't think so. (9)_____

P. I feel good as new. Thank you for all your help.

N. You're welcome. (10)_____

◇ Dialogue

Nurse:	It's time for your therapy, Mrs. Wati. I'll accompany you to the therapy room.
Mrs. Wati:	All right. I'll try using these crutches this time. Could you hand them to me?
Nurse:	Sure. Do you need help getting up?
Mrs. Wati:	No, I think I can do it.
Nurse:	That's it. Slowly.
Mrs. Wati:	*(Wincing.)* It's so hard.
Nurse:	You're almost there. I won't let you fall.
Mrs. Wati:	No, please don't touch me. Just give me a second to catch my breath.
Nurse:	Take your time. There's no hurry.
Mrs. Wati:	I've almost...got it...
Nurse:	You did it! Well done, Mrs. Wati. You're on your way to a full recovery.

Part Two Basic communication

Self-study sheet

Write the correct English sentences in the blanks. Learn them by heart!

1. ご気分はいかがですか．	
2. 何か持ってきましょうか．	
3. 心配しないで．大丈夫ですよ．	
4. 慌てないでください．	
5. お手伝いしましょうか．	
6. わかりました．	
7. 順調ですよ．	
8. きっとできますよ．	
9. もう一度やってみましょう．	
10. 続けてください．	
11. 完璧です．	
12. 少し休みましょうか．	
13. ちょっと顔色が悪いですね．	
14. 横になりたいのですか．	
15. しばらくおそばにいますよ．	
16. おつらいですね．	
17. 早く元気になるといいですね．	
18. 一番大変なところはもう終わりました．	
19. 安静が必要ですよ．	
20. お大事になさってください．	

Keep up the good work! 😊

Supplement
(Teacher's manual)

Extension task

Answers

Index

Extension Task

This book was designed to function both as a self-study workbook and as a primary textbook for a Nursing English course. An instructor using this book could follow the below lesson plan in a typical class.

> 1. **Vocabulary review/quiz.** Vocabulary and expressions from the previous chapter are reviewed. The instructor may also make a quiz sheet based on the previous chapter, and give this to students.
>
> 2. **Introduction of new vocabulary.** Students practice pronunciation of new words/expressions in the current chapter with the instructor.
>
> 3. **Exercises 1〜3.** This should be a partly oral task, with students reading sentences aloud in pairs as they complete the exercises. Time should be allowed for going over answers.
>
> 4. **Dialogue.** Students read the dialogue aloud in pairs, taking turns. The instructor may select some students to do a role play of parts or of the whole dialogue in groups or before the class.

For instructors who would like to include a communicative activity that requires collaboration and language production, we have included an **Extension Task** on the following page. Students, working in pairs, will write a short dialogue using at least two vocabulary or expressions from a target chapter. Students will practice reading this dialogue aloud, and then present it in groups or before the class.

If the instructor would like to use this activity on a weekly or regular basis, students can be instructed to write on their own papers.

本書は，看護英語コースの初級テキストとして，そして自学自習用にも使うことができるワークブックとして作成されています．講師の方は，標準的なクラスにおいて，次のような計画に従って授業を進めることができます．

1. 語彙の復習・クイズ　学習済みの章に登場した語彙や表現の復習．講師はクイズシートを作成し，学生のみなさんに配布するということもできます．
2. 新しい語彙の紹介　学生のみなさんは，講師に従って新しい章の単語・表現の発音練習ができます．
3. 練習問題1〜3　問題を終えたらペアになって文章を音読し，口頭での練習を盛り込むと効果的です．回答を考えるための十分な時間が必要です．
4. ダイアログ　学生さんがペアになり，交互に"Dialogue"を音読し，講師が数人の人を選び，グループごとに，またはクラスの前で，登場人物を割り振って練習する方法も良いでしょう．

共同作業や自ら言葉を考えることが必要な，コミュニケーションの要素を授業に取り入れたい講師の方々のために，次のページに「Extension Task」を掲載しておきます．ペアになった学生さんたちが，学習した章から2つ以上の語彙や表現を使って短い会話を作り，その音読練習をし，グループまたはクラスの前で発表できます．

もし，このようなレッスンを週に1回など定期的に行う場合は，学生さん各自のノートを活用してもらいましょう．

Extension task

Extension task

Part 1. *Write!* With a partner, write a short dialogue between a nurse and a patient (or between two nurses, or between a nurse and a doctor). Use your imagination! You only must use at least two vocabulary or expressions presented in this chapter. Write the dialogue in the box below.

Part 2. *Practice!* Read your dialogue aloud several times with your partner. Try to memorize it, and speak naturally.

Part 3. *Perform!* Some students will stand before the class and present their dialogue.

Have fun! 😀

Supplement

Answers

Chapter 1 Hospital departments and associated doctors
診療科と専門医

Exercise 1. 左の英語の語彙と右の日本語が一致するように選び，下の回答欄にアルファベットを記入しなさい．

1. b   2. f   3. g   4. d   5. h   6. j   7. i   8. e   9. c   10. a

Exercise 2. 下記の文を読んで，（　）内の正しい語彙に下線を引きなさい．設問 1 は回答例です．

1. 私の 5 歳の息子は（小児科 / pediatrics）に入院したばかりです．
2. 看護師のチャンさんは（精神科 / psychiatrics）に勤めています．
3. （婦人科医 / gynecologist）は女性の患者さんを診療します．
4. X 線撮影は，（放射線部 / radiology）へ行ってください．
5. ハリス医師は，（耳鼻咽喉科医 / otorhinolaryngologist）です．
6. （産科医 / obstetrician）は赤ちゃんを分娩させます．
7. 関口先生は，有名な（脳神経外科医 / neurosurgeon）です．
8. （麻酔科医 / anesthesiologist）は手術前にあなたを眠らせます．
9. （形成外科 / Reconstructive surgery）は 2 階にあります．
10. 主人は，明日（泌尿器科医 / urologist）の診察があります．

Exercise 3. 下の語彙表から適切な語彙を選び，文を完成させなさい．各語彙は 1 回のみ使用のこと．

1. 歯痛の場合，すぐに歯科医 / dentist の診察を受けてください．
2. 裕二さんは子どもが好きなので，小児 / pediatrics 看護師になりたいという希望を持っています．
3. 老年内科医 / geriatrician は，主にお年寄りを診療します．
4. 眼検査は，眼科 / ophthalmology へ行ってください．
5. 今インフルエンザが流行しているため，内科 / internal medicine 外来は混雑しています．
6. 山本さんは，足の骨折で 2 週間，整形外科 / orthopedics に入院しました．
7. 日焼けがひどいですね．皮膚科医 / dermatologist の診察をお勧めします．
8. 日本の病院では，産科医 / obstetricians が不足しています．
9. がん患者は，腫瘍内科 / oncology での診療が必要です．
10. 耳が痛いときは，耳鼻咽喉科医 / otorhinolaryngologist の診察をお勧めします．

Answers

◇ **Dialogue**

看護師　：　どうなさいましたか？

患　者　：　はい．皮膚科へはどう行ったらよいでしょうか？

看護師　：　それでしたら，この廊下をまっすぐ行きますと，右側にエレベータがあります．
　　　　　　皮膚科は3階です．エレベータを降りるとすぐ受付があります．

患　者　：　ありがとうございます．予約していないのですが，長く待つことになるでしょうか？

看護師　：　そんなに長くは待たないと思います．30分くらいでしょう．

患　者　：　そうですか．新聞や雑誌などがありますよね．

看護師　：　ございます．ただ，日本語のものばかりですが．

Self-study sheet
　空欄に正しい英語を記入しなさい．また，暗唱できるまで学習しなさい．

よくできました！ ☺

Supplement

Chapter 2 Healthcare personnel, patients, and other people
医療従事者と患者およびその関係者

Exercise 1. 左の英語の語彙と右の日本語が一致するように選び，下の回答欄にアルファベットを記入しなさい.

1. d　2. e　3. f　4. i　5. g　6. j　7. h　8. c　9. a　10. b

Exercise 2. 下記の文を読んで，（ ）内の正しい語彙に下線を引きなさい.

1. （放射線技師 / An X-ray technician）は放射線科で仕事をします.
2. 入り口の（受付係 / receptionist）で予約をしてください.
3. 病院で一夜過ごす人は，（入院患者 / inpatient）と呼ばれます.
4. （栄養士 / nutritionist）は，健康的な食事を選んでくれます.
5. （助産師 / midwife）は，分娩の手助けをしてくれます.
6. （手術室看護師 / surgical nurse）は，手術室で仕事をします.
7. （面会者 / Visitors）は，面会時間中に訪れるほうがよいでしょう.
8. （救急救命士 / EMTs）は，救急車で事故の現場に駆けつけます.
9. （薬剤師 / pharmacist）は薬を調剤してくれます.
10. （理学療法士 / physical therapist）は，歩行訓練をしてくれます.

Exercise 3. 下の語彙表から適切な語彙を選び，文を完成させなさい. 各語彙は1回のみ使用のこと.

1. 支払いは，1階の会計窓口係 / cashier でしてください.
2. 面会者 / Visitors は，患者さんの邪魔にならないように静かにしてください.
3. 歯科衛生士 / dental hygienist は，歯の掃除をします.
4. 食事に関しては，栄養士 / dietitian にご相談ください.
5. 最近，病院では看護師 / registered nurses が不足しています.
6. 理学療法士 / physical therapist は，筋力回復の指導をします.
7. この処方せんを薬剤師 / pharmacist にお渡しください.
8. 家庭で高齢者を介護するためには，もっと多くの介護福祉士 / care workers が必要とされます.
9. こちらのお子さまの保護者 / guardian の方ですか？
10. 宮武裕子です. この部署の看護師長 / head nurse をしています.

Answers

◇ **Dialogue**

患　者　：ほかに何をしたらよいでしょうか？

看護師　：まず，お支払いを済ませてください．1階の会計窓口係でこのファイルを提出してください．
　　　　　そのときに，保険証も提示してください．

患　者　：処方薬も院内でいただけますか？

看護師　：院外の薬局へ行ってください．当病院前にあります．受付係にこの処方せんをお渡しください．
　　　　　待ち時間はあまりないと思います．

患　者　：薬の内容を説明してもらえますか？

看護師　：してもらえますよ．理解できるまで，お尋ねください．

患　者　：お世話になりました．

看護師　：お大事に．

Self-study sheet
　空欄に正しい英語を記入しなさい．また，暗唱できるまで学習しなさい．

よかったですよ！ 😊

Supplement

Chapter 3 Medical supplies and equipment
医療用品と器具

Exercise 1. 左の英語の語彙と右の日本語が一致するように選び，下の回答欄にアルファベットを記入しなさい．

1. i   2. e   3. j   4. g   5. h   6. c   7. d   8. b   9. f   10. a

Exercise 2. 下記の文を読んで，（ ）内の正しい語彙に下線を引きなさい．

1. ご主人は自分で呼吸ができなくなっている状態ですから，（人工呼吸器 / <u>respirator</u>）を取り付けます．
2. 体重を測りますので，（体重計 / <u>scale</u>）に上がってください．
3. 放射線科に行きますので，（車椅子 / <u>wheelchair</u>）に乗ってください．
4. 傷口の（包帯 / <u>bandage</u>）を替えさせてください．
5. 腕の骨が折れていますから，約1ヵ月間（ギプス / <u>cast</u>）が必要です．
6. 深い傷ですね．傷口を閉じるために（縫合 / <u>stitches</u>）が必要です．
7. ドクターが舌に（舌圧子 / <u>tongue depressor</u>）をあてたら，"あー"と言ってください．
8. よくなっていますね．（歩行器 / <u>walker</u>）を使うと，上手に歩けるでしょう．
9. はっきり聞き取れなかったら，（補聴器 / <u>hearing aid</u>）を付けてください．
10. 医師が診察をしますので，（処置台 / <u>treatment table</u>）に仰向けになって寝てください．

Exercise 3. 下の語彙表から適切な語彙を選び，文を完成させなさい．各語彙は1回のみ使用のこと．

1. 車椅子 / <u>wheelchair</u> で手術室に行きましょう．
2. ギプス / <u>cast</u> が濡れないように，シャワーは浴びないでください．
3. 医師が，聴診器 / <u>stethoscope</u> で胸の音を聞きます．
4. 看護師さん，点滴の針 / <u>needle</u> のところが痛いです．
5. 傷を閉じるのに，5針の縫合 / <u>stitches</u> が必要です．
6. この吸入器 / <u>inhaler</u> を使用すれば，喘息の症状を抑えることができます．
7. 洗面器 / <u>washbasin</u> で顔は洗えますが，まだシャワーを浴びることはできません．
8. トイレに行きたくなったときには，便器 / <u>bedpan</u> を使用してください．
9. 血圧計 / <u>blood pressure gauge</u> で血圧を測ります．袖をまくってください．
10. 医師が，胃カメラ / <u>gastroscope</u> で胃の中を調べます．

Answers

◇ Dialogue

患　者　：ギプスはあとどのくらいつけていないといけませんか？

看護師　：少なくともあと1週間くらいはつけておいてもらわないといけないことになっています．

患　者　：目の上の糸（縫合）はどうですか？

看護師　：あと2～3日ですかね．

患　者　：よかった．かゆくて困っています．ギプスもできるだけ早くとれたらいいのになー．

看護師　：これだけは，骨がある程度固まるまで待ってもらわないといけませんね．そんなに長くないでしょう．

患　者　：そうですか．でも，もう我慢できないです．

看護師　：歩きたいのですね？

患　者　：またラグビーがしたいんです！

看護師　：もうしばらく休んでから，スポーツを始めてくださいね．

Self-study sheet

空欄に正しい英語を記入しなさい．また，暗唱できるまで学習しなさい．

素晴らしい！ 😊

Supplement

Chapter 4 Medication and treatment
薬剤と治療

Exercise 1． 左の英語の語彙と右の日本語が一致するように選び，下の回答欄にアルファベットを記入しなさい．

1. e   2. f   3. h   4. j   5. i   6. d   7. c   8. g   9. a   10. b

Exercise 2． 下記の文を読んで，（　）内の正しい語彙に下線を引きなさい．

1. ひどい頭痛です．（鎮痛剤 / <u>painkiller</u>）をもらえませんか．
2. この（軟膏 / <u>ointment</u>）を，1日2回やけどの箇所にぬってください．
3. アスピリンは，多くの国で一般的な（市販薬 / <u>over-the-counter medicine</u>）です．
4. この（睡眠剤 / <u>sleeping pill</u>）で，眠れるでしょう．
5. 大変な出血ですから，（輸血 / <u>a blood transfusion</u>）が必要でしょう．
6. （処方せん / <u>prescription</u>）を持って，1階の薬局に行ってください．
7. （使用説明 / <u>directions</u>）をしっかり守ってください．
8. この睡眠剤を（就寝時前 / <u>at bedtime</u>）に，飲んでください．
9. （投薬量 / <u>dosage</u>）は，患者の体の大きさと年齢によって異なります．
10. この（抗生物質 / <u>antibiotics</u>）を3日分出しておきます．

Exercise 3． 下の語彙表から適切な語彙を選び，文を完成させなさい．各語彙は1回のみ使用のこと．

1. サーチさんは腎不全のため，定期的に人工透析 / <u>dialysis</u> が必要です．
2. 1日2回，この白色で小さい方の錠剤 / <u>pill</u> を飲んでください．
3. 術後目覚めるまで，腕に点滴（静脈注射）/ <u>IV drip</u> をしておきます．
4. 多くの国で，臓器移植 / <u>organ transplantation</u> は，以前より普通に行われています．必要なら，新しい腎臓，心臓，それに肝臓なども入手できます．
5. 虫垂を切除するには，手術 / <u>operation</u> が必要となります．
6. 風邪の予防には，うがい薬 / <u>gargle</u> を何度も使用されるとよいでしょう．
7. 1日3回 食後 / <u>after meals</u>，抗生物質を服用してください．
8. この下剤 / <u>laxative</u> を服用すれば，トイレがもっと楽になります．
9. 経口 避妊薬 / <u>contraceptive</u> はコンドームの代用です．
10. また頭痛があれば，この鎮痛剤 / <u>painkiller</u> を服用してください．

Answers

◇ **Dialogue**

患　者　：この薬の服用法がわかりません．説明していただけませんか？

看護師　：はい．この大きな丸い錠剤は抗生剤です．1日3回 毎食後に服用してください．

患　者　：わかりました．

看護師　：この小さい楕円形の錠剤は鎮痛剤です．頭痛がひどいときだけ服用してください．

患　者　：空腹時でも服用できますか？

看護師　：できれば避けてください．何か食べてから服用してください．

　　　　　この散薬はかぜの症状を和らげます．朝と夕方の食後に服用してください．

患　者　：わかりづらいですね．覚えていられるかなー．

看護師　：大丈夫だとは思いますが，必ず指示に従ってくださいね．

Self-study sheet
　空欄に正しい英語を記入しなさい．また，暗唱できるまで学習しなさい．

これまでよく頑張りました！ ☺

Supplement

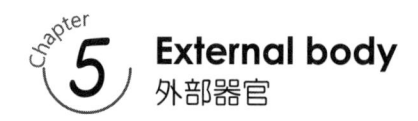

Chapter 5 External body
外部器官

Exercise 1. 左の英語の語彙と右の日本語が一致するように選び，下の回答欄にアルファベットを記入しなさい．

1. b 2. f 3. h 4. i 5. e 6. j 7. g 8. c 9. a 10. d

Exercise 2. 正しい語順に書き直した後，日本語で語彙を記述しなさい．設問1は回答例です．

1.	kcne	neck	頚部
2.	redluosh	shoulder	肩
3.	sbtutcok	buttocks	殿部
4.	preup mar	upper arm	上腕部
5.	weblo	elbow	肘部
6.	eto	toe	つま先
7.	slagetin	genitals	生殖器
8.	nisk	skin	皮膚
9.	iph	hip	股関節部
10.	pinlep	nipple	乳頭

Exercise 3. 下の語彙表から適切な語彙を選び，文を完成させなさい．各語彙は1回のみ使用のこと．

1. 彼は顔を殴られ，あご / jaw の骨を折りました．
2. ライナさんは転倒して，足関節 / ankle を捻挫しました．今あまり上手に歩けません．
3. あなたの皮膚 / skin の色は，とっても青白いです．夏には日焼け止めをつけるようにしてください．
4. あなたは，赤ちゃんを母乳で育てて / breast-feeding いますか？
5. 腕の下，脇窩 / armpit に体温計を挟んでください．
6. 仰向けになってください．医師が胸部 / chest の音を聞いてみます．
7. 肩 / shoulder を脱臼しましたね．しばらくの間，三角巾を使わないといけません．
8. フェルナンデスさんは，潰瘍のため腹部 / abdomen に焼けるような痛みを感じています．
9. これは大変，頬 / cheeks が赤くほてっていますね．熱がとっても高いですよ．
10. ジョン・スーンさんは，壊れたガラスを踏んで踵部 / heel を3針縫わなければなりませんでした．

Answers

◇ **Dialogue**

ハッサンさん ： 肩に痛みがあるので診察を受けたいのです．ひどい痛みです．

看　護　師 ： それは大変ですね．保険証をお持ちですか？

ハッサンさん ： 新しく仕事を始めたばかりで，まだもらっていません．国民健康保険には加入していますが…

看　護　師 ： 今の職場の電話番号を教えてください．

ハッサンさん ： すみませんが，わかりません．職場の人に話して，こちらへ電話してもらってもよいですか？

看　護　師 ： けっこうですが，できるだけ早く電話してくれるようにお伝えください．12:00 まで受け付けていますが，お昼は休みです．午後の診察時間は，2:30 から 6:00 までです．

ハッサンさん ： わかりました．ありがとうございます．

看　護　師 ： どういたしまして．

Self-study sheet
　　空欄に正しい英語を記入しなさい．また，暗唱できるまで学習しなさい．

だいぶよくなっていますよ！ ☺

Supplement

Chapter 6 Internal body I — Nervous, Sensory, Respiratory & Digestive system
内部器官 I — 脳神経系，感覚系，呼吸器系，消化器系

Exercise 1. 左の英語の語彙と右の日本語が一致するように選び，下の回答欄にアルファベットを記入しなさい．

1. c　2. h　3. g　4. j　5. e　6. d　7. f　8. b　9. i　10. a

Exercise 2. 欠落している部分に単語や文字を挿入し，語彙を完成させなさい．次に日本語の語彙も記入しなさい．

1. spinal cord　　　　　　脊髄
2. nasal cavity　　　　　　鼻腔
3. tympanic membrane　　鼓膜
4. voice box　　　　　　　喉頭
5. gallbladder　　　　　　 胆嚢
6. large intestine　　　　　大腸
7. vermiform appendix　　虫垂
8. windpipe　　　　　　　気管
9. esophagus　　　　　　 食道
10. rectum　　　　　　　　直腸

Exercise 3. 下の語彙表から適切な語彙を選び，文を完成させなさい．各語彙は1回のみ使用のこと．

1. ボリスさんはお酒を飲み過ぎて，肝臓 / liver がだいぶ弱っています．
2. のど / throat が赤くなっています．とっても痛そうです．
3. リンゴを食べているとき，スーザンさんは誤って舌 / tongue をかみました．
4. 咽頭炎は咽頭 / pharynx の痛みを伴う炎症です．
5. 健康診断のため尿と便 / stool を持ってきてください．
6. ペトラさんは脊髄 / spinal cord を損傷して，下半身不随です．
7. 喫煙は肺 / lung がんの原因となります．
8. 牡蠣を食べてから，胃 / stomach 痛があります．
9. 肉をとりすぎる食事は，結腸 / colon がんの原因となります．
10. 自転車用ヘルメットは，脳 / brain の損傷を防止します．

Answers

◇ **Dialogue**

看護師　：これは胃内視鏡検査の説明書です．前日の午後 9:00 以降は絶食です．
　　　　　0:00 以降は何も飲まないでください．

患　者　：朝，歯磨きをしてもよいですか？

看護師　：かまいませんが，水は飲みこまないようにしてください．
　　　　　それから，少しゆったりしたものを着てください．

患　者　：運転してきてよいでしょうか．

看護師　：歩くか，誰かに乗せてきてもらうほうがよいでしょう．
　　　　　麻酔後，自動車や自転車に乗るのは危険です．

患　者　：麻酔は痛いですか？　心配です．

看護師　：気分が多少悪くなるでしょうが，それほどではないと思います．
　　　　　胃の状態がわかるベストな方法ですから．

Self-study sheet
　空欄に正しい英語を記入しなさい．また，暗唱できるまで学習しなさい．

このまま頑張って！ ☺

Supplement

Chapter 7 Internal body II Circulatory, Blood and Immune, Endocrine, Reproductive & Urogenital system
内部器官II — 循環器系，血液・免疫系，内分泌系，泌尿・生殖器系

Exercise 1. 左の英語の語彙と右の日本語が一致するように選び，下の回答欄にアルファベットを記入しなさい．

1. d   2. b   3. i   4. f   5. e   6. j   7. g   8. c   9. a   10. h

Exercise 2. 欠落している部分に単語や文字を挿入し，語彙を完成させなさい．次に日本語の語彙も記入しなさい．

1. bone marrow — 骨髄
2. prostate — 前立腺
3. lymph node — リンパ節
4. thyroid gland — 甲状腺
5. urinary bladder — 膀胱
6. erythrocyte — 赤血球
7. white blood cell — 白血球
8. uterus — 子宮
9. kidney — 腎臓
10. cervix — 子宮頚管

Exercise 3. 下の語彙表から適切な語彙を選び，文を完成させなさい．各語彙は1回のみ使用のこと．

1. 看護師さん，尿 / urine がうまく出なくて困っているのですが．
2. 看護師さんは私の静脈 / vein をうまく見つけられなくて困っています．減量をしたほうがいいですね．
3. erythrocyte（ギリシャ語由来の医学用語）の一般用語は，赤血球 / red blood cell です．
4. 白血球 / white blood cell 数が高いのは，感染症の徴候かもしれません．
5. 子宮 / uterus の壁に，腫瘍があります．
6. 前立腺 / Prostate がんは，50歳以上の男性に顕著にみられます．
7. 脾臓 / spleen は，古くなった赤血球を排泄します．
8. 尿管 / ureter は尿を腎臓から膀胱へ運ぶ管です．
9. 主人は，精子 / sperm 数が少ないです．
10. セルジさんは胸にひどい痛みを感じ，以前に心臓 / heart 発作を患っていると診断されました．

Answers

◇ **Dialogue**

女性(母)　：　すみませんが，息子の血液検査の結果を説明していただけませんか？　まだよくわかりません．

看　護　師　：　これが白血球数です．とても高いので，息子さんは，まだ尿管感染が続いていると思われます．

女性(母)　：　先生は，なぜこの数字をマルで囲んだのでしょうか？

看　護　師　：　これは血中の鉄分の数値です．とっても低いですね．貧血の可能性があります．

女性(母)　：　先生がそう言っていました．それであの茶色の薬を服用しなければならないのですね．

看　護　師　：　そうです．鉄分は肺に酸素を運ぶのに必要ですが，それが欠乏しているので息子さんは疲れやすいのです．

女性(母)　：　レバーのような鉄分が豊富な食事をすればよいのですか？

看　護　師　：　それでもよいのですが，鉄分のサプリも摂取してください．

女性(母)　：　それは，深刻ですね．せめてわかっただけでも救われます．ありがとうございました．

Self-study sheet
　　空欄に正しい英語を記入しなさい．また，暗唱できるまで学習しなさい．

完璧！ ☺

Chapter 8 Musculoskeletal system
筋骨格系

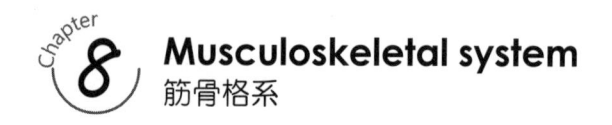

Exercise 1. 左の英語の語彙と右の日本語が一致するように選び，下の回答欄にアルファベットを記入しなさい．

1. g   2. c   3. j   4. d   5. i   6. f   7. a   8. h   9. e   10. b

Exercise 2. 表の空白箇所に適切な語彙を記入し完成させなさい．1問目は回答例です．

	Medical word	Common word	日本語
1.	cranium	skull	頭蓋骨
2.	maxilla	upper jaw	上顎骨
3.	mandible	lower jaw	下顎骨
4.	clavicle	collar bone	鎖骨
5.	scapula	shoulder blade	肩甲骨
6.	spine	backbone	脊椎
7.	sternum	breastbone	胸骨
8.	patella	kneecap	膝蓋骨
9.	carpus	wrist bone	手根骨
10.	tibia	shin bone	脛骨
11.	femur	thigh bone	大腿骨

Exercise 3. 下の語彙表から適切な語彙を選び，文を完成させなさい．各語彙は1回のみ使用のこと．

1. パークさんは頭を打って，頭蓋骨 / skull を骨折しました．
2. 大腿骨 / femur は，ヒトの体で一番強固な骨です．
3. カタリナさんは，昨年鎖骨 / collar bone を骨折して，今でもときどき肩に痛みを感じます．
4. フットボールをプレイ中に胸を打って，2本の肋骨 / ribs にひびが入りました．
5. 井上さんは，右前腕の尺骨 / ulna を折りました．
6. ボルキさんは，ちょうど肘の上の上腕骨 / humerus を折りました．
7. 手首の靭帯 / ligament が切れているようです．手術で治す必要があります．
8. 過度な運動をすると，筋肉 / muscles を傷めます．
9. タラドクさんは，座るたびに尾骨 / tail bone に痛みを感じます．
10. 幸いにも，あなたのおばあさまは転倒したときに骨盤 / pelvis を骨折しませんでした．

Answers

◇ **Dialogue**

看 護 師　：ゴムリッチさん，今日の膝の具合はいかがですか？

ゴムリッチさん：ずきんずきんしますが，昨日よりだいぶよくなりました．

看 護 師　：そうですか．靭帯は手術できれいに治っていますから，あとは回復を待つだけでしょう．

ゴムリッチさん：足の骨も痛いです．ここです．

看 護 師　：それは，脛骨にボルトを入れたから痛いのです．来週は松葉杖を使って，膝に体重があまりかからないようにしてください．

ゴムリッチさん：リハビリ（理学療法）はいつから始まりますか？

看 護 師　：じつは，今からリハビリにお連れします．よろしいですか？

ゴムリッチさん：待っていました！

看 護 師　：その気ですよ！　もうすぐ歩けますよ．

Self-study sheet
　空欄に正しい英語を記入しなさい．また，暗唱できるまで学習しなさい．

さらに頑張れ！ ☺

Supplement

Chapter 9 — Illnesses and conditions I
Nervous; Ear, Nose, Throat and Eye; Respiratory; Digestive; Blood and Immune; and Endocrine systems

病気と症状 I ― 脳神経系，耳鼻咽喉系，呼吸器系，消化器系，血液・免疫系，内分泌系

Exercise 1. 左の英語の語彙と右の日本語が一致するように選び，下の回答欄にアルファベットを記入しなさい．

1. g　2. f　3. i　4. e　5. j　6. d　7. a　8. c　9. h　10. b

Exercise 2. 欠落している部分に単語や文字を挿入し，語彙を完成させなさい．次に日本語の語彙も記入しなさい．

1. laryngitis　　　　　　　喉頭炎
2. deafness　　　　　　　聴覚障害
3. cirrhosis of the liver　　肝硬変
4. food poisoning　　　　食中毒
5. stomach ulcer　　　　胃潰瘍
6. tuberculosis　　　　　結核
7. diabetes mellitus　　　糖尿病
8. anemia　　　　　　　　貧血
9. pneumonia　　　　　　肺炎
10. cerebrovascular accident　脳卒中

Exercise 3. 下の語彙表から適切な語彙を選び，文を完成させなさい．各語彙は1回のみ使用のこと．

1. お子さんは専門用語でotitis mediaといいますが，中耳炎 / middle ear infection にかかっています．痛みが伴います．
2. 大きな虫歯 / cavity があります．来週先生が治療いたします．
3. 毎春，花粉症 / hay fever になります．目がかゆくて困ります．
4. お嬢さんの喘息 / asthma 発作のときに，この吸入器を使えば楽になります．
5. 肺がん / lung cancer の一般に考えられる原因の一つは喫煙です．
6. リンさんは，白血病 / leukemia で治療中です．頭の毛も抜け落ちました．
7. 田中さんは，よく片頭痛 / migraine があります．
8. 糖尿病 / diabetes の場合，血糖値をチェックすることが大切です．
9. 脳卒中 / stroke 以来，祖父は話しをするのが困難になりました．
10. チェンさん，あまり心配することはないですよ．かぜ / common cold ですから．

Answers

◇ **Dialogue**

イトウさん ： 娘は熱が高く，咳が止まりません．ミルクも少しも飲んでいないし，痛みもひどいようです．

看護師 ： そうですか．体温を測ってください．

イトウさん ： 測りました．40度くらいでした．今すぐ先生にみてもらえますか？

看護師 ： できるだけ早くみてもらいましょう．ほかにも患者さんがいらっしゃいますので，もう少しお待ち下さい．

イトウさん ： 肺炎かもしれません．急を要します．私の国では，重症患者は優先的にみてもらえます．

看護師 ： 申し訳ありませんが，順番が来るまでお待ち下さい．もう一度体温を測ってくださいませんか？処置には，できるだけ詳しい状態を知ったほうがよいと思います．

Self-study sheet
　　空欄に正しい英語を記入しなさい．また，暗唱できるまで学習しなさい．

半分終わりましたよ！ ☺

Supplement

Chapter 10 Illnesses and conditions II — Circulatory; Urogenital; Musculoskeletal; Skin; Mental; and Other systems
病気と症状 II ― 循環器系，泌尿・生殖器系，筋骨格系，皮膚系，精神系，その他

Exercise 1. 左の英語の語彙と右の日本語が一致するように選び，下の回答欄にアルファベットを記入しなさい．

1. d 2. b 3. f 4. i 5. e 6. j 7. h 8. g 9. c 10. a

Exercise 2. 欠落している部分に単語を挿入し，語彙を完成させなさい．次に日本語の語彙も記入しなさい．

1. enlarged prostate　　　　前立腺肥大症
2. renal failure　　　　　　腎不全
3. Down syndrome　　　　ダウン症候群
4. acne vulgaris　　　　　にきび
5. cold sore　　　　　　　疱疹
6. urinary tract infection　尿路感染症
7. myocardial infarction　　心臓発作
8. hardening of the arteries　動脈硬化症
9. infectious disease　　　感染症
10. athlete's foot　　　　　水虫，足白癬

Exercise 3. 下の語彙表から適切な語彙を選び，文を完成させなさい．各語彙は1回のみ使用のこと．

1. 祖母は認知症 / dementia です．私の名前も覚えていません．
2. 肥満 / Obesity は，食事療法と運動で抑制できます．
3. 水虫（足白癬）/ fungal infection ですから，お子さんと一緒の入浴を控えたほうがよいでしょう．
4. 鋭い胸の痛みは，心臓発作 / heart attack の可能性があります．
5. このこぶのようなものは，いぼ / warts です．液体窒素で処置します．
6. リウマチ / Rhematism は，心臓や骨，関節，肺，それに腎臓疾患などを引き起こすことになります．
7. 顔の吹き出物はニキビ / acne の徴候です．
8. 強迫性障害は，一種の神経症 / neurosis です．
9. 食事の減塩することは，高血圧 / hypertension の治療に効果があります．
10. 足の親指のはれは，痛風 / gout です．

◇ Dialogue

ハッドソンさんは前立腺肥大症の手術をし，回復を待って入院中です．

看　護　師　：ハッドソンさん，単刀直入にお聞きしますが，今日何度おしっこされましたか？

ハッドソンさん　：2回です．

看　護　師　：そのとき痛みとか，不快感はありませんでしたか？

ハッドソンさん　：少しはありましたが，昨日よりは軽いです．

看　護　師　：今回は，血尿がありましたか？

ハッドソンさん　：はい，まだ少し茶色がかっていました．

看　護　師　：朝，便は出ましたか？

ハッドソンさん　：はい，朝起きてからすぐにありました．

看　護　師　：やわらかい便でしたか，それとも硬かったですか？

ハッドソンさん　：ちょうど中間くらいでした．普通だと思います．

Self-study sheet

空欄に正しい英語を記入しなさい．また，暗唱できるまで学習しなさい．

その調子！ 😊

Supplement

Chapter 11 Children's and women's illnesses and conditions
小児・婦人科の疾患と症状

Exercise 1. 左の英語の語彙と右の日本語が一致するように選び，下の回答欄にアルファベットを記入しなさい．

1. g   2. b   3. a   4. h   5. d   6. e   7. j   8. i   9. f   10. c

Exercise 2. 欠落している部分に語彙や文字を挿入し，語彙を完成させなさい．次に日本語の語彙も記入しなさい．

1. menopausal <u>disorder</u>　　　　　更年期障害
2. extrauterine <u>pregnancy</u>　　　　子宮外妊娠
3. heavy <u>menstrual</u> periods　　　　月経過多
4. post-<u>partum</u> depression　　　　産後うつ病
5. <u>whooping</u> cough　　　　　　　百日咳
6. sudden infant death <u>syndrome</u>　乳幼児突然死症候群
7. yeast <u>infection</u>　　　　　　　　カンジダ症
8. <u>pink</u> eye　　　　　　　　　　　結膜炎
9. <u>uterine</u> myoma　　　　　　　　子宮筋腫
10. chickenpo<u>x</u>　　　　　　　　　　水痘

Exercise 3. 下の語彙表から適切な語彙を選び，文を完成させなさい．

1. <u>注意欠陥多動性障害 / ADHD</u> の子どもたちは，学校で注意力が散漫になりやすいです．
2. <u>つわり / Morning sickness</u> により，妊娠の最初2〜3ヵ月はとてもつらい期間です．
3. <u>陣痛 / contractions</u> が始まったら，すぐ病院へ来てください．
4. 初めて親になった方にとって，<u>乳幼児突然死症候群 / SIDS</u> はとても心配ですが，それはまれなことです．
5. 咳をしたときの引きつけは，<u>百日咳 / pertussis</u> の徴候です．
6. このかゆいところは，<u>水痘 / chickenpox</u> の徴候です．しかし，鶏肉を食べてなるようなものではありません．
7. ご主人は，<u>出産 / delivery</u> に立ち会われますか．
8. <u>風疹 / German measles</u> は，ドイツ人の医師によって初めて報告されました．
9. ひどい摂食障害の女性は，<u>無月経 / absence of periods</u> を経験するかもしれません．
10. <u>卵巣がん / Ovarian cancer</u> は，女性の「サイレントキラー（沈黙の殺人者）」と呼ばれます．

Answers

◇ **Dialogue**

張さん ： 看護師さん，娘のことが心配です．黄疸は重症ですよね．

看護師 ： 心配はいりません．新生児の場合，黄疸は，特にアジアではよくみられます．
お子さんは，血中に黄色色素が少し多めにみられるだけですから．

張さん ： でも，ドクターが言うには，脳を損傷することも考えられるとのことですが．主人と私は心配で，
病気になりそうです．

看護師 ： それは，まれなケースですから．光線療法を1日受けられると元気になりますよ．

張さん ： でも，光線療法を受けなければならない（幼い）娘を見るだけでも，かわいそうでなりません．
娘に触ることさえできないでしょう．この処置は心理的な後遺症の原因となりませんか？

看護師 ： 絶対なりませんから．すぐお嬢さんを抱っこできます．私の言うことを信じてください．

Self-study sheet
空欄に正しい英語を記入しなさい．また，暗唱できるまで学習しなさい．

ここからは下り坂です！ ☺

101

Supplement

Chapter 12 Injuries and emergencies
外傷と救急

Exercise 1. 左の英語の語彙と右の日本語が一致するように選び，下の回答欄にアルファベットを記入しなさい．

1. c 2. e 3. g 4. i 5. a 6. f 7. h 8. j 9. d 10. b

Exercise 2. 正しい語順に並べかえ，下線上に文章として書きなさい．

1. Her leg muscles cramped while swimming. — 彼女の足の筋肉は，水泳中にこむら返りを起こしました．
2. She is having a seizure. — 彼女は，今ひきつけを起こしています．
3. He fell and scraped his knee. — 彼は転倒し，膝に擦過傷を負いました．
4. He lost consciousness two hours ago. — 彼は，2 時間前に気を失いました．
5. She found a lump in her breast. — 彼女は，胸にしこりを見つけました．
6. He nearly drowned in the river. — 彼は危うく溺死するところでした．
7. Your father is paralyzed. — あなたのお父さまが全身不随になりました．
8. He has a concussion. — 彼は脳しんとう状態にあります．
9. You have sprained your ankle. — あなたは，足首を捻挫しています．
10. Your wrist is broken. — あなたの手首は骨折しています．

Exercise 3. 下の語彙表から動詞または前置詞を選び，空白箇所に記入しなさい．

1. Her arm <u>was</u> badly wounded in the traffic accident. — 彼女は，交通事故で腕をひどく損傷しました．
2. I <u>have</u> painful blisters on my feet. — 足に痛い水泡 / 水ぶくれがあります．
3. Don't be alarmed, but I have <u>found</u> a tiny lump in your breast. — 聞いて心配しないでね，胸にしこりが見つかりました．
4. I'm afraid that this cut will <u>leave</u> a scar. — 申し訳ありませんが，この切り傷の跡は残るでしょう．
5. Your grandmother is <u>in</u> a coma now. — おばあさまは今昏睡状態にあります．
6. The EMTs <u>administered</u> CPR but could not revive the man. — 救急医療班（EMTs）は，心肺蘇生法を施しましたが，男性を生き返らせることはできませんでした．
7. Edgar has been <u>on</u> artificial respiration for three days. — エドガーは 3 日間人工呼吸を施されていました．
8. Xian <u>attempted</u> suicide by mixing dangerous chemicals. — シアンさんは，危険な化学物質を混ぜ合わせて自殺を企てました．
9. Her forearms <u>were</u> lacerated by a man with a knife. — 彼女は，ナイフを持った男から前腕を切りつけられました．
10. Your mother has <u>lost</u> consciousness again. — お母さまがまた意識を失いました．

Answers

◇ Dialogue

ピミエントさんは自転車から落ちて，救急病棟に来ました．

看　護　師　：ピミエントさん，膝にひどいすり傷を負いましたね．でも，思ったよりひどくないようで，不幸中の幸いですね．

ピミエントさん　：そうです．日本で自転車に乗るのは不慣れでして．

看　護　師　：今から傷口を消毒して，小石やごみを取り出しますね．

ピミエントさん　：そうですか．痛そう．

看　護　師　：ちょっとチクッとしますが，すぐ終わります．足を伸ばしてくださいませんか．痛いときはすぐに言ってください．

（看護師が傷口をきれいにする．）

看　護　師　：はい，もう終わりましたよ．そんなに痛くなかったでしょう？

ピミエントさん　：痛くはなかったけれど，チクッとしました．傷跡は残りますか？

看　護　師　：残らないでしょう．きれいに治りますから．

Self-study sheet

空欄に正しい英語を記入しなさい．また，暗唱できるまで学習しなさい．

素晴らしいできばえです！☺

Supplement

Chapter 13 Common complaints
主訴

Exercise 1. 左の英語の語彙と右の日本語が一致するように選び，下の回答欄にアルファベットを記入しなさい．

1. _b_ 2. _i_ 3. _a_ 4. _j_ 5. _d_ 6. _f_ 7. _e_ 8. _k_ 9. _c_ 10. _g_

Exercise 2. 下記の文を読んで，（ ）内の正しい語彙に下線を引きなさい．また完成した文を右に書きなさい．

1.	racing	My heart is racing.	脈が速くなっています．
2.	worried	I'm worried about this rash.	この発疹が気になっています．
3.	sweat	I sweat a lot at night.	寝汗がひどいです．
4.	hurts	It hurts when I breathe.	息をすると胸が痛みます．
5.	sneezing	I have sneezing fits all day.	一日中，くしゃみが出ます．
6.	cough	I have a dry cough.	かわいた咳が出ます．
7.	stuffed up	My nose is all stuffed up.	鼻が詰まっています．
8.	splitting	I have a splitting headache.	頭が割れそうに痛みます．
9.	myself	I haven't been myself lately.	最近調子が悪いです．
10.	sluggish	I feel so sluggish.	体がだるいです．

Exercise 3. 下の語彙表から適切な語彙を選び，文を完成させなさい．

N. What seems to be the problem? — どうなさいましたか？

P. It (1) <u>hurts</u> when I breathe and I've been coughing up (2) <u>phlegm</u>. — 息をすると胸が痛みます．咳をすると痰も出ます．

N. Do you have any other symptoms? — ほかにどのような症状がありますか？

P. Yes. I (3) <u>vomited</u> twice this morning. — そうですね．今朝2回吐きました．

N. Do you feel (4) <u>feverish</u>? — 体が熱っぽいですか？

P. Yes, I'm hot, and I'm (5) <u>constipated</u>, too. My bowels haven't moved for three days. — 熱いです．便秘もしています．3日ほど便が出ません．

N. What seems to be the trouble? — どうなさいましたか．

P. I have a (6) <u>runny</u> nose and I've had (7) <u>sneezing</u> fits all day. And I have a (8) <u>sore</u> throat. — 一日中，鼻水とくしゃみが出ています．喉も痛いです．

N. Hmm. You're running a low-grade fever, too. Anything else? — そうですね，微熱もありますね．ほかには？

P. My eyes are (9) <u>itchy</u> and I have a (10) <u>pounding</u> headache. It's like someone is hitting my head with a hammer. I'm just in bad shape! — 目がかゆいです．それに，頭がずきずき痛みます．ハンマーで頭を叩かれているようです．どうしようもない状態です．

注）pounding =（何かに叩かれるように）ずきずきする．splitting = 割れそうな．ここでは pounding が適当．

Answers

◇ **Dialogue**

看 護 師 ： 初診の患者様には，この用紙をご記入いただいております．お名前，住所，電話番号，生年月日をお書きいただけますか？ ローマ字で結構です．

（記入が終わってから）

看 護 師 ： それでは，どうされましたか？

ウエイさん ： はい，咳が止まらないので来ました．止まりそうもありません．それに，鼻水も出ます．

看 護 師 ： 鼻水はどんな色をしていますか？

ウエイさん ： 黄色がかった色です．感染しているのでしょうか？

看 護 師 ： ドクターがお答えできると思います．名前が呼ばれるまでこちらに座ってお待ちください．

Self-study sheet
　空欄に正しい英語を記入しなさい．また，暗唱できるまで学習しなさい．

大変よくできました！ 😊

Supplement

Chapter 14 Taking a patient's history
病歴の聴取

Exercise 1. 左の英文と右の日本語の表現が一致するように選び，下の回答欄にアルファベットを記入しなさい．

1. b   2. d   3. c   4. a   5. i   6. e   7. h   8. f   9. g   10. j

Exercise 2. 左右の句を適切に組み合わせ，下線上に完成した文章を書きなさい．

1. f   Are you allergic to any medications? 　薬に対するアレルギーはありますか．
2. c   How long have you had this fever? 　熱はどのくらい続いていましたか．
3. i   Do you exercise regularly? 　定期的に運動しますか．
4. b   Do you have any chronic illnesses? 　慢性の病気はありますか．
5. h   Has anyone in your family been hospitalized for a serious illness? 　ご家族の中に大きな病気で入院された方はいらっしゃいますか．
6. j   How many times do you urinate in a day? 　排尿は1日に何回ありますか．
7. g   Have you ever had a serious illness before? 　これまでに大きな病気をしたことがありますか．
8. d   Are you sleeping well? 　よく眠れますか．
9. e   What is your occupation? 　ご職業は何ですか．
10. a   Are your periods regular? 　月経は規則正しくありますか．

Exercise 3. 患者さんの返答から看護師の質問を考え，それを下線上に書きなさい．

N. (1) Do you have any chronic illnesses? 　慢性の病気はありますか．
P. Chronic? Well, I had asthma when I was a child, but now I'm fine. 　慢性の？　そうですね，子どものころは喘息もちでしたが，今はだいじょうぶです．

N. (2) Have you ever had a serious illness before? 　これまでに大きな病気をしたことがありますか．
P. Yes, I had pneumonia two or three times as a child. Nothing more serious than that, though. 　はい，子どものころ，2〜3回肺炎にかかりました．そのくらいです．

N. (3) Is there a history of heart problems in your family? 　ご家族の中で心臓病にかかったことがある方はいらっしゃいますか．
P. Yes, my father and grandfather both had heart problems. 　はい，父と祖父が心臓病でした．

N. (4) Do you smoke? 　タバコを吸いますか．
P. Yes. I do. I smoke a pack a day. 　はい．1日1箱吸います．

Answers

N. (5) <u>How is your appetite?</u>   食欲はありますか．
P. Just fine. In fact I'm hungry now.   はい．今もおなかがすいていますし．

N. (6) <u>Do you exercise regularly?</u>   定期的に運動しますか．
P. Not regularly, but I sometimes cycle to work.   定期的ではないですが，ときどき自転車通勤します．

N. (7) <u>Do you have any allergies?</u>   何かアレルギーはありますか．
P. Yes, I'm allergic to house dust and mold.   はい，ハウスダストとカビのアレルギーです．

N. (8) <u>Are you taking any medication now?</u>   何か薬を飲んでいますか．
P. Yes, I take some medicine to control my allergies.   はい，アレルギーの薬を数種類飲んでいます．

N. (9) <u>Are your periods regular?</u>   月経は規則正しくありますか．
P. Yes, they are. Every 29 days.   はい．29日ごとです．

N. (10) <u>When was your last period?</u>   最終月経はいつでしたか．
P. Last week.   先週です．

◇ Dialogue

マクダーモットさんは，年に一度の定期健康診断を受けています．

看　護　師　：日常の生活様式についての質問をしますが，よろしいでしょうか．
マクダーモットさん：どうぞ，よろしくお願いします．
看　護　師　：最初に，タバコを吸いますか？
マクダーモットさん：いいえ．今まで一度も吸ったことはありません．
看　護　師　：お酒などは飲みますか？
マクダーモットさん：はい，たしなみます．
看　護　師　：1日にどのくらい飲まれますか？
マクダーモットさん：毎日ではないです．飲むとしたら大半が週末です．
看　護　師　：どんなお酒で，量はどのくらいですか？
マクダーモットさん：もっぱらビールです．毎回1～2缶くらいです．

Self-study sheet

空欄に正しい英語を記入しなさい．また，暗唱できるまで学習しなさい．

だいぶ進歩しましたよ！ ☺

Supplement

Chapter 15 Giving instructions during an examination
検査時の助言

Exercise 1. 左の英文と右の日本語の表現が一致するように選び，下の回答欄にアルファベットを記入しなさい．

1. _b_   2. _c_   3. _f_   4. _d_   5. _i_   6. _h_   7. _g_   8. _j_   9. _e_   10. _a_

Exercise 2. 左右の句を適切に組み合わせ，下線上に完成した文章を書きなさい．

1. _f_   I'm going to take a blood sample.   採血します．
2. _a_   Please roll up your sleeve.   腕をまくってください．
3. _j_   Please give me your right arm.   右手を出してください．
4. _b_   This may prick a little.   チクッとしますよ．
5. _g_   Please fill this cup about one-third full.   カップの 1/3 まで尿を入れてください．
6. _h_   Please take off your shirt.   上着を脱いでください．
7. _d_   Breathe in and out slowly.   ゆっくり息を吸ったり吐いたりしてください．
8. _e_   Please lie down on the bed.   ベッドに横になってください．
9. _c_   Please roll over onto your stomach.   うつ伏せになってください．
10. _i_   You can sit up now.   どうぞ起き上がってください．

Exercise 3. 患者さんの返答から看護師の質問を考え，それを下線上に書きなさい．各会話は質問と返答で完結し，長い連続した会話ではない．

N. (1) I'm going to take a blood sample.　　　　　　　　　採血します．
P. Blood sample? All right, but I really hate needles.　　採血？ わかりました，針はきらいなのですが．

N. (2) Please fill this cup about one-third full.　　　　　　カップの 1/3 まで尿を入れてください．
P. About one-third, OK. Where should I put this cup when I finish?　　1/3 くらいですね．終わったら，カップはどこへ置けばいいですか？

N. (3) Please roll up your sleeve.　　　　　　　　　　　袖をまくってください．
P. OK. Is it rolled up far enough?　　　　　　　　　　はい．かなり上までまくるのですか？

N. (4) Please wait in front of the examination room.　　　　検査室の前でお待ち下さい．
P. All right. Will I have to wait long for the doctor?　　　はい．長く待たなくてはいけませんか？

N. (5) Please lie down on the bed.　　　　　　　　　　　ベッドに横になってください．
P. Should I take off my shoes before lying down?　　　　靴をぬいだほうがいいですか？

N.	(6) <u>Please give me your right arm.</u>	右手を出してください．
P.	I'd prefer my left, actually.	左のほうがいいのですが．
N.	(7) <u>We're going to take a chest X-ray.</u>	胸の写真をとります．
P.	I really don't like X-rays.	X線は好きではありません．
N.	(8) <u>Please keep this thermometer under your arm until it beeps.</u>	ピーと鳴るまで体温計を腋の下にはさんでおいてください．
P.	(*Pause*). I don't think this is working. I didn't hear any beep.	（じっと待つ）これは動作していないと思います．何の音も聞こえませんでした．
N.	(9) <u>Hold still for a moment.</u>	しばらく動かないでください．
P.	I am holding still.	じっとしています．
N.	(10) <u>Please take off your shirt.</u>	上着を脱いでください．
P.	Do I have to take off my t-shirt, too?	Tシャツも脱いだほうがいいですか？

◇ Dialogue

看　護　師　： 身長と体重をはかります．靴を脱いで，この体重計に上がってください．

トーマスさん　： はい．

看　護　師　： 71.5キロです．今度は身長です．この台の上に上がってください．背中をまっすぐにしてください．それでけっこうです．165センチですね．今度はここに座って，名前を呼ばれるまでお待ちください．

（数分後）

看　護　師　： トーマスさん，どうぞお入りください．ここにお座りください．どちらの腕にしますか？

トーマスさん　： 右腕にします．

看　護　師　： 袖をまくってください．楽にしてください．チクッとしますよ．
はい，終わりました．これをもう少し押さえておいてくださいね．けっこうですよ．
もう一度待合室でお待ちください．20分くらい経ってからお帰りください．

Self-study sheet

空欄に正しい英語を記入しなさい．また，暗唱できるまで学習しなさい．

上手にできましたよ！ ☺

Supplement

Chapter 16. Common questions from foreign patients
外国人患者がよく問う質問

Exercise 1. 左の英文と右の日本語の表現が一致するように選び，下の回答欄にアルファベットを記入しなさい．

1. _e_ 2. _a_ 3. _j_ 4. _b_ 5. _c_ 6. _g_ 7. _d_ 8. _i_ 9. _h_ 10. _f_

Exercise 2. 質問に必要な語彙を記入し，下記の下線上に完成した文章を書きなさい．

1. _Is_   Is the X-ray machine safe?   X線は安全ですか．
2. _How_   How many days do I have to be hospitalized?   入院は何日間ぐらいですか．
3. _Does_   Does this medicine have any side effects?   この薬に何か副作用はありますか．
4. _Where_ Where should I keep my valuables?   貴重品はどこに置けばいいですか．
5. _Does_   Does this meal contain pork?   この食事には豚肉が入っていますか．
6. _When_   When will the test results be ready?   検査の結果はいつわかりますか．
7. _Could_ Could you please stay with me?   私のそばにいてくれませんか．
8. _Will_   Will the operation be painful?   手術は痛みますか．
9. _What_   What does this medicine do?   この薬は何のためですか．
10. _How_   How long will this IV take?   点滴はどのくらい時間がかかりますか．

Exercise 3. 看護師の返答から患者さん質問を考え，それを下線上に書きなさい．各会話は質問と返答で完結し，長い連続した会話ではない．

P. (1) I'm feeling better. Can I check out early?   だいぶ良くなりました．早く退院してもいいですか．
N. I'm sorry but it is still too soon for you to check out.   申し訳ありませんが，退院するにはまだ早すぎると思われます．

P. (2) Will I be awake during the operation?   手術中は目が覚めていますか．
N. No, you will be asleep during the operation.   いいえ，手術中はぐっすり眠っています．

P. (3) When will the test result be ready?   検査の結果はいつわかりますか．
N. They'll be ready in about an hour.   1時間ほどです．

P. (4) How many days do I have to be hospitalized?   入院は何日間くらいですか．
N. You will need to be here for about two or three days.   2〜3日の入院が必要でしょう．

P. (5) What do I need to bring with me when I'm hospitalized?   入院するときに必要な持ち物は何ですか．
N. Pajamas, a towel, underwear, eating utensils and toiletries.   パジャマ，タオル，下着，食器や箸など，それに洗面用具などです．

Answers

P. (6) <u>How did the operation go?</u>　　　　　　手術はうまくいきましたか．
N. It went very well.　　　　　　　　　　　　　すべてうまくいきました．

P. (7) <u>Can I be transferred to a private room?</u>　個室に移りたいです．
N. I'm sorry, none are available now.　　　　　　申し訳ありませんが，今，空いている個室はありません．

P. (8) <u>Can I see the doctor now?</u>　　　　　　　今 主治医に会えますか．
N. The doctor is doing his rounds now but will be back in the afternoon.　　今 回診中ですが，午後には戻られます．

P. (9) <u>This medicine isn't working. Can you change it?</u>　この薬は効きません．変えてもらえませんか．
N. It may take a little time for the medicine to work. Please be patient.　　薬が効いてくるのに多少時間がかかります．どうぞ辛抱強くお待ちください．

P. (10) <u>Is it OK if I eat before the operation?</u>　手術の前に食べてもいいですか．
N. No, you shouldn't eat anything on the day of the operation.　　手術の当日は，絶食です．

◇ Dialogue

患　者　：前に見たことのないような薬ですが，どのように飲んだらよいのですか？

看護師　：粉薬です．包みを開けて，口に入れて，コップ1杯の水で一気に飲み込んでください．

患　者　：わかりました．3日分の処方しかありませんね．1週間分もらえませんか？

看護師　：申し訳ありません．医師が，3日分しか出しておりませんから．

患　者　：3日してもまだよくならない場合はどうしたらよいですか？　もう少し出してほしいのですが．

看護師　：3日後に薬が効かないようであれば，ほかの薬を出しますから，もう一度おいでください．それでいかがでしょうか？

患　者　：はい，わかりました．それから，先生が febrile（熱 fever の形容詞形で，熱のあること）とおっしゃっていました．不安です．それはどういうことですか．

看護師　：単に熱があるということです．何も不安になることではありませんから．

Self-study sheet
　空欄に正しい英語を記入しなさい．また，暗唱できるまで学習しなさい．

もう少しで終わりですよ！

Supplement

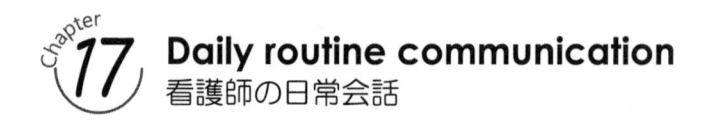

Chapter 17　Daily routine communication
看護師の日常会話

Exercise 1. 左の英文と右の日本語の表現が一致するように選び，下の回答欄にアルファベットを記入しなさい．

1. _g_　2. _h_　3. _a_　4. _e_　5. _j_　6. _b_　7. _i_　8. _c_　9. _d_　10. _f_

Exercise 2. 正しい語順に並べかえ，下線上に文章として書きなさい．

1.	I'll be your primary nurse.	担当看護師です．
2.	I'm sorry to disturb your rest.	お休み中すみません．
3.	You need your own towel and toiletries.	タオルや洗面用具はご自分でご用意ください．
4.	Please let me know if you feel any pain.	痛みがあれば言ってください．
5.	I'm sorry to have kept you waiting.	お待たせしました．
6.	How was your meal?	食事はどうでしたか．
7.	Visiting hours are over.	面会時間は終わりました．
8.	Press the call button if you need anything.	もし何かあればナースコールを押してください．
9.	Could you please speak more slowly?	もう少しゆっくり話してください．
10.	Do you have a health insurance card?	保険証はお持ちですか．

Exercise 3. 患者さんの返答・質問から看護師の言葉を考え，それを下線上に書きなさい．各会話は質問と返答で完結し，長い連続した会話ではない．

N.	(1) Excuse me. May I come in?	失礼します．
P.	Sure, come in.	どうぞお入りください．
N.	(2) Please do not use your cellular phone in this room.	この部屋では携帯電話を使わないでください．
P.	Well, where can I use it then?	では，どこで使用できますか．
N.	(3) Did you take your medicine?	薬は飲まれましたか．
P.	Oops, I forgot. I'll take it now.	しまった，忘れていました．今飲みますから．
N.	(4) Do you have any questions?	何かご質問はありますか．
P.	Not right now. You've explained everything very well.	今のところはありません．よく説明していただきましたから．
N.	(5) Are you familiar with procedures in a Japanese hospital?	日本の病院の手続きなどはおわかりですか．
P.	Yes, I think so. This is my third time to stay in a Japanese hospital.	はい，なんとか．日本の病院に入院するのはこれで3度目ですから．

Answers

P. I'm worried about the food here. — どうもここでの食べ物が心配なのですが．

N. Hmm. (6) <u>Are there any foods that you cannot eat?</u> — そうですか．食べられないものはありますか．

P. What should I do with this tray when I'm done eating? — 食べ終わったら，このトレイはどうしたらよいですか．

N. (7) <u>Please return your tray to the cart after you've finished.</u> — 食べ終わったら，トレイをカートにお返しください．

P. I feel really grubby. When can I take a bath? — 体が汚れている感じですが，いつお風呂に入れますか．

N. (8) <u>You may take a bath from 8:00am to 8:00pm.</u> — お風呂は午前 8:00 から午後 8:00 まで入れます．

P. Nurse, I have a question about (*mumble*). — 看護師さん，（ぼそぼそ言う）についてお聞きしたいのですが．

N. (9) <u>Pardon me?</u> または <u>Could you repeat that?</u> — もう一度言ってください．

P. I can't speak Japanese. Does anyone on staff speak English? — 日本語を話せませんが，どなたか英語のできる方はいらっしゃいますか．

N. (10) <u>I can speak a little English.</u> — 私は少し英語を話せます．

◇ Dialogue

看 護 師 ： オウルさん，体温を測る時間です．昼食はどうでしたか？

オウルさん ： おいしかったですよ．朝食よりはずっとましでした．

看 護 師 ： どのくらい食べられましたか？

オウルさん ： 全部食べました．まだ食べたいくらいです．

看 護 師 食欲はよいとしても，まだ熱がありますね．

オウルさん ： 気分はよいので，できたら病院の外を散歩したい気持ちです．
外の空気を吸って，元気になりたいです．

看 護 師 ： 医師に聞いてみますが，もう少し休んだほうがよろしいですよ．
院内で歩き回ってみてはいかがですか？

オウルさん そうですか．では，もう1日待ってみます．

注）会話で，"not bad, not so bad, not too bad" は，「なかなかよい，かなりよい」の意味で使われる．

Self-study sheet

空欄に正しい英語を記入しなさい．また，暗唱できるまで学習しなさい．

素晴らしいできばえです！ ☺

Supplement

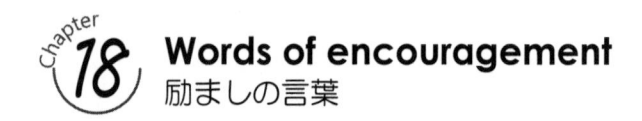

Chapter 18 Words of encouragement
励ましの言葉

Exercise 1. 左の英文と右の日本語の表現が一致するように選び，下の回答欄にアルファベットを記入しなさい．

1. b   2. f   3. g   4. j   5. c   6. i   7. d   8. e   9. a   10. h

Exercise 2. 左右の句を適切に組み合わせ，下線上に完成した文章を書きなさい．

1. d   Can I get you anything?　　　　　　　　　　何か持ってきましょうか．
2. a   There's no need to panic.　　　　　　　　　慌てないでください．
3. f   I'm sure you can do it.　　　　　　　　　　きっとできますよ．
4. g   Shall we take a break?　　　　　　　　　　少し休みましょうか．
5. h   You're doing great.　　　　　　　　　　　　順調ですよ．
6. i   You need to get some rest.　　　　　　　　安静が必要ですよ．
7. e   Let's give it another try.　　　　　　　　　もう一度やってみましょう．
8. c   You look a bit pale.　　　　　　　　　　　ちょっと顔色が悪いですね．
9. j   The worst is behind you.　　　　　　　　　一番大変なところはもう終わりました．
10. b   This must be very difficult for you.　　　　おつらいですね．

Exercise 3. 患者さんの返答・質問から看護師の言葉を考え，それを下線上に書きなさい．各会話は質問と返答で完結し，長い連続した会話ではない．

N. (1) How are you feeling?　　　　　　　　　　　　ご気分はいかがですか．
P. I'm feeling much better, thanks.　　　　　　　　おかげさまで，とっても気分がよいです．

N. (2) I'll stay with you for a while.　　　　　　　しばらくおそばにいますよ．
P. Thanks for staying. I appreciate your company.　ありがとう．一緒にいてもらえて感謝します．

N. (3) You look a bit pale.　　　　　　　　　　　　ちょっと顔色が悪いですね．
P. Pale? Well, I feel like I might vomit.　　　　　顔色が悪いですって．今にも吐きそうな気分です．

N. (4) Shall we take a break?　　　　　　　　　　　少し休みましょうか．
P. Good idea. I could use a break.　　　　　　　　そうしましょう．休憩もよいね．

N. (5) Let's give it another try.　　　　　　　　　もう一度やってみましょう．
P. O.K. I'll give it another shot.　　　　　　　　よーし．やってみようか．

P. I think I need some help getting out of bed.　　ベッドから出るのに助けがいるかもしれません．
N. (6) Here, let me help you.　　　　　　　　　　　お手伝いしましょう．

114

Answers

P. My son is allergic to dairy products. 　息子は，乳製品アレルギーなのですが．

N. (7) <u>I understand.</u> または <u>I see.</u> He'll have special non-dairy meals. 　わかりました．特別に乳製品以外の食事をご用意しましょう．

P. I'm a little worried about the operation tomorrow. 　明日の手術のことですが，心配です．

N. (8) <u>Don't worry. Everything will be fine.</u> 　心配しないで．大丈夫ですよ．

P. Today's therapy was really hard. Will it be as hard tomorrow? 　今日の治療は本当に大変でした．明日も同じようでしょうか．

N. I don't think so. (9) <u>The worst is behind you now.</u> 　そうではないと思いますよ．一番大変なところはもう終わりました．

P. I feel good as new. Thank you for all your help. 　生まれ変わったようです．大変お世話になりました．

N. You're welcome. (10) <u>Please take care of yourself.</u> 　どういたしまして．お大事になさってください．

◇ Dialogue

看 護 師 ： ワティさん，治療の時間です．治療室まで一緒に行きます．

ワティさん ： よろしくお願いします．松葉杖で行きたいのですが，取ってもらえますか．

看 護 師 ： はい．自分で立てますか．

ワティさん ： できます．

看 護 師 ： はい．ゆっくり，ゆっくり．

ワティさん ： （痛みをこらえながら）つらいねー．

看 護 師 ： もうそこです．お手伝いしましょうか．

ワティさん ： 触らないで．息を吸ってからまた続けますから．

看 護 師 ： ゆっくりね．急がなくてもよいですよ．

ワティさん ： もう少し，もう少し…

看 護 師 ： とうとう着いたね．やったわね，ワティさん．もう回復に向かっているわね．

Self-study sheet

空欄に正しい英語を記入しなさい．また，暗唱できるまで学習しなさい．

これからも頑張ってください！ ☺

Index

英和
(Ch.=Chapter)

abdomen 腹部 (Ch.5)
absence ないこと，欠如，*absence of periods* 無月経 (Ch.11)
acne にきび (Ch.10)
acne vulgaris にきび (Ch.10)
acute poliomyelitis 急性灰白髄炎，ポリオ (Ch.11)
after meals 食後 (Ch.4)
allergic アレルギーの (Ch.14)
allergy アレルギー (Ch.14)
amenorrhea 無月経 (Ch.11)
analgesic 鎮痛剤 (Ch.4)
anemia 貧血 (Ch.9)
anesthesiologist 麻酔科医 (Ch.1)
anesthesiology 麻酔科 (Ch.1)
ankle 足関節 (Ch.5)
antibiotic(s) 抗菌薬，抗生物質 (Ch.4)
appendix 虫垂 (Ch.6)
appetite 食欲 (Ch.14)
arm 腕，手 (Ch.15)
armpit 腋窩 (Ch.5)
arteriosclerosis 動脈硬化症 (Ch.10)
artery 動脈 (Ch.7)
arthritis 関節炎 (Ch.10)
artificial respiration 人工呼吸 (Ch.12)
asphyxiation 窒息 (Ch.12)
asthma 喘息 (Ch.9)
at bedtime 就寝時前，眠前 (Ch.4)
athlete's foot 水虫，足白癬 (Ch.10)
attempt suicide 自殺を図る (Ch.12)
attending physician 主治医 (Ch.2)
attention deficit hyperactivity disorder (ADHD) 注意欠陥多動性障害 (Ch.11)
autism 自閉症 (Ch.10)
awake 目が覚めている (Ch.16)
axilla 腋窩 (Ch.5)
backbone 脊椎，脊柱 (Ch.8)
bandage 包帯 (Ch.3)
bath お風呂 (Ch.17)
bedpan 便器 (Ch.3)
bladder 膀胱 (Ch.7)
blindness 視覚障害 (Ch.9)
blister 水疱 (Ch.12)
blood pressure 血圧 (Ch.15)
blood pressure gauge 血圧計 (Ch.3)
blood sample 血液検体，*take a blood sample* 採血する (Ch.15)
blood transfusion 輸血 (Ch.4)
bone 骨 (Ch.8)
bone marrow 骨髄 (Ch.7)
bowel 腸，*regular bowel movements* 規則正しい便通 (Ch.14)
bra ブラジャー (Ch.15)
brain 脳 (Ch.6)
break 休憩 (Ch.18)
breast 乳房 (Ch.5)
breast cancer 乳がん (Ch.11)
breastbone 胸骨 (Ch.8)
breath 息 (Ch.15)
breathe 息をする (Ch.13)
broken bone 骨折 (Ch.12)
bronchitis 気管支炎 (Ch.9)
bruise 打撲傷 (Ch.12)
burn 熱傷 (Ch.12)
buttocks 殿部，尻 (Ch.5)
call button ナースコールボタン (Ch.17)
candidiasis カンジダ症 (Ch.11)
cardiologist 循環器内科医 (Ch.1)
cardiology 循環器内科 (Ch.1)
cardiopulmonary resuscitation (CPR) 心肺蘇生法 (Ch.12)
care 保護，世話，*take care of yourself* お大事に (Ch.18)
care giver 介護福祉士 (Ch.2)
care worker 介護福祉士 (Ch.2)
carpus 手根骨 (Ch.8)
cart カート (Ch.17)
cartilage 軟骨 (Ch.8)
cashier 会計窓口係 (Ch.2)
cast ギプス (Ch.3)
cavity う蝕，虫歯 (Ch.9)
cellular phone 携帯電話 (Ch.17)
cerebrovascular accident (CVA) 脳卒中 (Ch.9)
cervical cancer 子宮頚がん (Ch.11)
cervix 子宮頚管 (Ch.7)
change 変える (Ch.16)
check out 退院する (Ch.16)
check out procedures 退院手続き (Ch.16)
cheek 頬部，頬 (Ch.5)
chest 胸部 (Ch.5)
chest X-ray 胸部X線 (Ch.15)
chickenpox 水痘 (Ch.11)
children's doctor 小児科医 (Ch.1)
chin 頤 (Ch.5)
choke 詰まらせる (Ch.12)
chronic illness 慢性疾患 (Ch.10, 14)
cigarette タバコ (Ch.14)
cirrhosis of the liver 肝硬変 (Ch.9)
clavicle 鎖骨 (Ch.8)
clinic 医院，診療所 (Ch.17)
clinical depression うつ病 (Ch.10)
clinical psychologist 臨床心理士 (Ch.2)
clinical resident 研修医 (Ch.2)
clothes 衣服 (Ch.16)
coccyx 尾骨 (Ch.8)
cold sore 疱疹 (Ch.10)
collar bone 鎖骨 (Ch.8)
colon 結腸 (Ch.6)
coma 昏睡状態 (Ch.12)
comatose 昏睡状態の (Ch.12)
common cold かぜ，感冒 (Ch.9)
community health nurse 保健師 (Ch.2)
concern 心配事 (Ch.17)
concussion 脳しんとう (Ch.12)
conjunctivitis 結膜炎 (Ch.11)
constipate 便秘をさせる (Ch.13)
contain 入れている，含む (Ch.16)
contraceptive 避妊薬 (Ch.4)
contractions 陣痛 (Ch.11)
cough medicine 鎮咳剤 (Ch.4)
cough suppressant 鎮咳剤 (Ch.4)
cramp こむら返り (Ch.12)
cranium 頭蓋骨 (Ch.8)
crutch 松葉杖 (Ch.3)
cut 創傷，傷 (Ch.12)
cystitis 膀胱炎 (Ch.11)
deafness 聴覚障害 (Ch.9)
delivery 分娩 (Ch.11)
dementia 認知症 (Ch.10)
dental caries う蝕，虫歯 (Ch.9)
dental hygienist 歯科衛生士 (Ch.2)
dentist 歯科医 (Ch.1)
dentistry 歯科 (Ch.1)
dermatologist 皮膚科医 (Ch.1)
dermatology 皮膚科 (Ch.1)
diabetes 糖尿病 (Ch.9)
diabetes mellitus (DM) 糖尿病 (Ch.9)
dialysis 人工透析 (Ch.4)
diaphragm 横隔膜 (Ch.6)
diarrhea 下痢 (Ch.13)
dietitian 栄養士 (Ch.2)
difficult 困難な，つらい (Ch.18)
directions 使用説明 (Ch.4)
discomfort 不快な感じ (Ch.17)
disinfectant 消毒液 (Ch.3)
dislocation 脱臼 (Ch.12)
disturb 妨げる，じゃまをする (Ch.17)
dizzy 立ちくらみ（めまい）がする (Ch.13)
doctor 医師 (Ch.2, 16)
dosage 投薬量 (Ch.4)

Index

dose　投薬量　(Ch.4)
Down syndrome　ダウン症候群　(Ch.10)
drown　溺水する　(Ch.12)
dry cough　かわいた咳　(Ch.13)
dull　調子が悪い，だるい　(Ch.13)
earache　耳痛，耳の痛み　(Ch.13)
eardrum　鼓膜　(Ch.6)
eat　食べる　(Ch.17)
ectopic pregnancy　子宮外妊娠　(Ch.11)
elbow　肘部，肘　(Ch.5)
EMT (Emergency Medical Technician)　救命救急士　(Ch.2)
endocrinologist　内分泌科医　(Ch.1)
endocrinology　内分泌科　(Ch.1)
endoscope　内視鏡　(Ch.3)
enlarged prostate　前立腺肥大症　(Ch.10)
ENT (Ear, Nose and Throat) doctor　耳鼻咽喉科医　(Ch.1)
erythrocyte　赤血球　(Ch.7)
esophagus　食道　(Ch.6)
examination room　検査室　(Ch.15)
exercise　運動する　(Ch.14)
explain　説明する，教える　(Ch.16)
extrauterine pregnancy　子宮外妊娠　(Ch.11)
eye doctor　眼科医　(Ch.1)
fatigue　疲れ，だるさ　(Ch.13)
feces　便　(Ch.6)
feel　感じる，気分（ここち）を感じる　(Ch.18)
femur　大腿骨　(Ch.8)
fever　熱　(Ch.14)
feverish　熱っぽい　(Ch.13)
fibula　腓骨　(Ch.8)
fine　申し分ない，すばらしい　(Ch.18)
fist　握りこぶし　(Ch.15)
food　食べ物　(Ch.17)
food poisoning　食中毒　(Ch.9)
forearm　前腕部　(Ch.5)
forehead　前額部　(Ch.5)
fracture　骨折　(Ch.12)
fungal infection　水虫，足白癬　(Ch.10)
gallbladder　胆嚢　(Ch.6)
gargle　含そう剤，うがい薬　(Ch.4)
gastritis　胃炎　(Ch.9)
gastroenterologist　消化器内科医　(Ch.1)
gastroenterology　消化器内科　(Ch.1)
gastroscope　胃カメラ　(Ch.3)
gauze　ガーゼ　(Ch.3)
genitals　生殖器　(Ch.5)
geriatrician　老年内科医　(Ch.1)
geriatrics　老年内科　(Ch.1)

German measles　風疹　(Ch.11)
gingiva　歯肉　(Ch.6)
gout　痛風　(Ch.10)
great　うまく，じょうずな　(Ch.18)
guardian　保護者　(Ch.2)
gum　歯肉　(Ch.6)
gynecologist　婦人科医　(Ch.1)
gynecology　婦人科　(Ch.1)
hallux　つま先　(Ch.5)
hardening of the arteries　動脈硬化症　(Ch.10)
hay fever　花粉症　(Ch.9)
head nurse　病棟師長　(Ch.2)
health insurance card　保険証　(Ch.17)
hearing aid　補聴器　(Ch.3)
heart　心臓　(Ch.7)
heart attack　心臓発作　(Ch.10)
heart problem　心臓病　(Ch.14)
heat stroke　熱中症　(Ch.10)
heavy menstrual periods　月経過多　(Ch.11)
heel　踵部　(Ch.5)
height scale　身長計　(Ch.3)
help　手伝う　(Ch.18)
hemorrhoids　痔核　(Ch.9)
hepatic cirrhosis　肝硬変　(Ch.9)
hepatitis　肝炎　(Ch.9)
herbal medicine　漢方薬　(Ch.4)
herpes simplex　単純疱疹　(Ch.10)
high blood fat　高脂血症　(Ch.10)
high blood pressure (HBP)　高血圧　(Ch.10)
hip　股関節部，腰周り　(Ch.5)
hold still　動かないでいる，じっとしている　(Ch.15)
hora somni (h.s.)　就寝時前，眠前　(Ch.4)
hospital　病院　(Ch.17)
hospitalize　入院させる　(Ch.14)
hot　熱い　(Ch.13)
humerus　上腕骨　(Ch.8)
hurt　痛む　(Ch.13)
hyperlipidemia　高脂血症　(Ch.10)
hypertension　高血圧　(Ch.10)
hypothermia　低体温　(Ch.12)
infectious disease　感染症　(Ch.10)
inhaler　吸入器　(Ch.3)
injury　けが　(Ch.12)
inpatient　入院患者　(Ch.2)
insomnia　不眠症　(Ch.10)
internal medicine　内科　(Ch.1)
internist　内科医　(Ch.1)
itchy　かゆい　(Ch.13)
IV (intravenous)　点滴　(Ch.16)

IV drip　点滴静脈注射　(Ch.4)
IV pole　点滴棒　(Ch.3)
IV stand　点滴スタンド　(Ch.3)
jaundice　黄疸　(Ch.11)
jaw　あご　(Ch.5)
job　職業　(Ch.14)
joint　関節　(Ch.8)
keep　続ける，*keep going*　続ける，進み続ける　(Ch.18)
kidney　腎臓　(Ch.7)
kidney failure　腎不全　(Ch.10)
knee　膝　(Ch.5)
kneecap　膝蓋骨　(Ch.8)
labor pains　陣痛　(Ch.11)
laceration　裂傷　(Ch.12)
large intestine　大腸　(Ch.6)
laryngitis　喉頭炎　(Ch.9)
larynx　喉頭　(Ch.6)
laxative　下剤　(Ch.4)
leukemia　白血病　(Ch.9)
leukocyte　白血球　(Ch.7)
lie down　横になる　(Ch.15, 18)
ligament　靭帯　(Ch.8)
liquid medicine　水薬　(Ch.4)
liver　肝臓　(Ch.6)
lower jaw　下顎骨　(Ch.8)
lump　腫瘤，しこり　(Ch.12)
lung　肺　(Ch.6)
lung cancer　肺がん　(Ch.9)
lung carcinoma　肺がん　(Ch.9)
lymph node　リンパ節　(Ch.7)
mandible　下顎骨　(Ch.8)
manometer　血圧計　(Ch.3)
marry　結婚する　(Ch.14)
maxilla　上顎骨　(Ch.8)
meal　食事　(Ch.16, 17)
measles　麻疹　(Ch.11)
meat　肉　(Ch.16)
medication　薬　(Ch.14)
medicine　薬　(Ch.16, 17)
meningitis　髄膜炎　(Ch.9)
menopausal disorder　更年期障害　(Ch.11)
menorrhagia　月経過多　(Ch.11)
middle ear infection　中耳炎　(Ch.9)
midwife　助産師　(Ch.2)
migraine　片頭痛　(Ch.9)
miscarriage　流産　(Ch.11)
morning sickness　つわり，妊娠悪阻　(Ch.11)
mouthwash　含そう剤，うがい薬　(Ch.4)
mumps　流行性耳下腺炎　(Ch.11)
muscle　筋肉　(Ch.8)
muteness　言語・音声障害　(Ch.9)

117

Supplement

myocardial infarction (MI)　心筋梗塞 (Ch.10)
myself　自分自身, *I haven't been myself lately.* 調子が悪い (Ch.13)
nail　爪 (Ch.5)
nasal cavity　鼻腔 (Ch.6)
nausea and vomiting during pregnancy (NVP)　つわり, 妊娠悪阻 (Ch.11)
nauseous　吐き気がする (Ch.13)
neck　頚部, 首 (Ch.5)
needle　針 (Ch.3)
nerve　神経 (Ch.6)
nervous　心配な, 不安な, 緊張している (Ch.16)
neurologist　神経内科医 (Ch.1)
neurology　神経内科 (Ch.1)
neurosis　神経症 (Ch.10)
neurosurgeon　脳神経外科医 (Ch.1)
neurosurgery　脳神経外科 (Ch.1)
nipple　乳頭 (Ch.5)
nutritionist　栄養士 (Ch.2)
obesity　肥満 (Ch.10)
obstetrician　産科医 (Ch.1)
obstetrics　産科 (Ch.1)
occupation　職業 (Ch.14)
ointment　軟膏 (Ch.4)
once a day　1日1回 (Ch.4)
oncologist　腫瘍内科医 (Ch.1)
oncology　腫瘍内科 (Ch.1)
operation　手術 (Ch.4, 16)
ophthalmologist　眼科医 (Ch.1)
ophthalmology　眼科 (Ch.1)
organ transplantation　臓器移植 (Ch.4)
orthopedics　整形外科 (Ch.1)
orthopedist　整形外科医 (Ch.1)
otitis media　中耳炎 (Ch.9)
otolaryngologist　耳鼻咽喉科医 (Ch.1)
otolaryngology　耳鼻咽喉科 (Ch.1)
otorhinolaryngologist　耳鼻咽喉科医 (Ch.1)
otorhinolaryngology　耳鼻咽喉科 (Ch.1)
outpatient　外来患者 (Ch.2)
ovarian cancer　卵巣がん (Ch.11)
ovary　卵巣 (Ch.7)
over-the-counter medicine (OTC medicine)　市販薬 (Ch.4)
pain　痛み (Ch.17)
painful　痛い (Ch.16)
painkiller　鎮痛剤 (Ch.4)
pale　青白い, 蒼白な (Ch.18)
pancreas　膵臓 (Ch.6)
panic　慌てる (Ch.18)
paralysis　麻痺 (Ch.12)
pardon　*Pardon me?* もう一度言ってください (Ch.17)
parotitis　流行性耳下腺炎 (Ch.11)
patella　膝蓋骨 (Ch.8)
pediatrician　小児科医 (Ch.1)
pediatrics　小児科 (Ch.1)
pelvis　骨盤 (Ch.8)
penis　陰茎 (Ch.7)
perfect　完璧な (Ch.18)
period　(月経などの) 周期, *last period* 最終月経 (Ch.13)
perspire　汗をかく (Ch.13)
pertussis　百日咳 (Ch.11)
pharmacist　薬剤師 (Ch.2)
pharynx　咽頭 (Ch.6)
phlegm　痰 (Ch.13)
physical therapist　理学療法士 (Ch.2)
physician　医師, 内科医 (Ch.1, 2)
piles　痔核 (Ch.9)
pill　錠剤 (Ch.4)
pink eye　結膜炎 (Ch.11)
placenta　胎盤 (Ch.7)
plasma　血漿 (Ch.7)
plastic surgeon　形成外科医 (Ch.1)
plastic surgery　形成外科 (Ch.1)
pneumonia　肺炎 (Ch.9)
polio　急性灰白髄炎, ポリオ (Ch.11)
pollinosis　花粉症 (Ch.9)
pork　豚肉 (Ch.16)
post cibum (p.c.)　食後 (Ch.4)
post-partum depression　産後うつ病 (Ch.11)
pounding (headache)　ずきずきする (頭痛) (Ch.13)
powdered medicine　散剤 (Ch.4)
practitioner　医師 (Ch.2)
prescribe　処方する (Ch.4)
prescription　処方せん (Ch.4)
press　押す (Ch.17)
prick　チクッと痛ませる (Ch.15)
primary nurse　担当看護師 (Ch.17)
private room　個室 (Ch.16)
procedure　手続き (Ch.16, 17)
productive cough　痰を伴った咳 (Ch.13)
prostate　前立腺 (Ch.7)
prostatomegaly　前立腺肥大症 (Ch.10)
psychiatrics　精神科 (Ch.1)
psychiatrist　精神科医 (Ch.1)
pulmonologist　呼吸器内科医 (Ch.1)
pulmonology　呼吸器内科 (Ch.1)
quaque die (q.d.)　1日1回 (Ch.4)
question　質問 (Ch.17)
race　(脈などが) 走る, 速くなる (Ch.13)
radiologist　放射線科医 (Ch.1)
radiology　放射線科 (Ch.1)
radius　橈骨 (Ch.8)
rash　発疹 (Ch.13)
receptionist　受付係 (Ch.2)
reconstructive surgery　形成外科 (Ch.1)
rectum　直腸 (Ch.6)
red blood cell　赤血球 (Ch.7)
registered nurse (RN)　看護師 (Ch.2)
regular　規則正しい (Ch.14)
regularly　定期的に, 規則正しく (Ch.14)
relax　力をぬく (Ch.15)
renal failure　腎不全 (Ch.10)
repeat　繰り返して言う (Ch.17)
resident　研修医 (Ch.2)
respirator　人工呼吸器 (Ch.3)
rest　休憩, 睡眠 (Ch.17, 18)
return　返す, 返却する, 戻す (Ch.17)
rheumatism　リウマチ (Ch.10)
rib　肋骨 (Ch.8)
roll over　寝返りをうつ, *roll over onto one's stomach* うつ伏せになる (Ch.15)
roll up　(袖などを) まくる (Ch.15)
rubella　風疹 (Ch.11)
rubeola　麻疹 (Ch.11)
run　*the runs* 下痢 (Ch.13)
runny nose　鼻水 (Ch.13)
safe　安全な (Ch.16)
salve　軟膏 (Ch.4)
scale　*weight scale* 体重計, *height scale* 身長計 (Ch.3)
scapula　肩甲骨 (Ch.8)
scar　傷跡 (Ch.12)
scrape　擦過傷 (Ch.12)
scrub nurse　手術室看護師 (Ch.2)
see　わかる, 理解する, *I see.* (Ch.18)
seizure　痙攣 (Ch.12)
senility　認知症 (Ch.10)
serious illness　大きな病気, 重い病気 (Ch.14)
sexually transmitted disease (STD)　性感染症 (Ch.10)
shin bone　脛骨 (Ch.8)
shirt　シャツ, 上着 (Ch.15)
short of breath　息切れ (Ch.13)
shoulder　肩 (Ch.5)
shoulder blade　肩甲骨 (Ch.8)
shower　シャワー (Ch.16)
side effect　副作用 (Ch.16)
sink　洗面器 (Ch.3)
sit up　起き上がる (Ch.15)
skin　皮膚 (Ch.5)

Index

skin doctor 皮膚科医 (Ch.1)
skull 頭蓋骨 (Ch.8)
sleep 眠る (Ch.13)
sleeping pill 睡眠剤 (Ch.4)
sleeve 袖 (Ch.15)
sling 三角巾 (Ch.3)
slowly ゆっくり (Ch.15, 17)
sluggish 調子が悪い，だるい (Ch.13)
small intestine 小腸 (Ch.6)
smoke タバコを吸う (Ch.14)
sneezing fits くしゃみの発作，止まらないくしゃみ (Ch.13)
sore 痛い (Ch.13)
sorry すまないと思う (Ch.17)
speak 話す (Ch.17)
sperm 精子 (Ch.7)
sphygmomanometer 血圧計 (Ch.3)
spinal cord 脊髄 (Ch.6)
spine 脊椎，脊柱 (Ch.8)
spleen 脾臓 (Ch.7)
splitting (headache) 割れそうな (頭痛) (Ch.13)
spontaneous abortion 流産 (Ch.11)
sprain 捻挫 (Ch.12)
stay いる，とどまる，*stay with* 〜 〜と一緒にいる，〜のそばにいる (Ch.16, 18)
sternum 胸骨 (Ch.8)
stethoscope 聴診器 (Ch.3)
stitches 縫合 (Ch.3)
stomach 胃 (Ch.6)
stomach ache 胃炎 (Ch.9)
stomach ulcer 胃潰瘍 (Ch.9)
stool 便 (Ch.6)
stress ストレス (Ch.14)
stretcher ストレッチャー (Ch.3)
stroke 脳卒中 (Ch.9)
stuffed up （鼻などが）詰まっている (Ch.13)
sudden infant death syndrome (SIDS) 乳幼児突然死症候群 (Ch.11)
suffocation 窒息 (Ch.12)
suicide 自殺 (Ch.12)
sunstroke 熱中症 (Ch.10)

supplement サプリメント (Ch.14)
suppository 坐薬 (Ch.4)
surgery 手術 (Ch.4)
surgical nurse 手術室看護師 (Ch.2)
sutures 縫合 (Ch.3)
sweat 汗をかく (Ch.13)
syringe 注射器 (Ch.3)
tail bone 尾骨 (Ch.8)
tendon 腱 (Ch.8)
test 検査 (Ch.16)
test results 検査結果 (Ch.16)
testicle 精巣 (Ch.7)
thermometer 体温計 (Ch.15)
thigh 大腿部 (Ch.5)
thigh bone 大腿骨 (Ch.8)
thirsty 喉が渇いている (Ch.13)
throat 咽喉 (Ch.6)
thyroid gland 甲状腺 (Ch.7)
tibia 脛骨 (Ch.8)
tire 疲れ（させる）(Ch.13)
toe つま先 (Ch.5)
toiletry 洗面用具 (Ch.17)
tongue 舌 (Ch.6)
tongue depressor 舌圧子 (Ch.3)
tonsil 扁桃腺 (Ch.6)
towel タオル (Ch.17)
trachea 気管 (Ch.6)
transfer 移る，移す (Ch.16)
tray トレイ (Ch.17)
treatment table 処置台 (Ch.3)
try 試み，努力，*give it another try* もう一度やってみる (Ch.18)
t-shirt T-シャツ (Ch.15)
tuberculosis (TB) 結核 (Ch.9)
tympanic membrane 鼓膜 (Ch.6)
ulna 尺骨 (Ch.8)
unconscious 意識不明 (Ch.12)
understand わかる，理解する (Ch.18)
upper arm 上腕部 (Ch.5)
upper jaw 上顎骨 (Ch.8)
ureter 尿管 (Ch.7)
urethra 尿道 (Ch.7)
urinary bladder 膀胱 (Ch.7)

urinary tract infection (UTI) 尿路感染症 (Ch.10)
urinate 排尿する (Ch.14)
urine 尿 (Ch.7)
urine sample 尿検体 (Ch.15)
urologist 泌尿器科医 (Ch.1)
urology 泌尿器科 (Ch.1)
use 使う (Ch.17)
uterine fibroids 子宮筋腫 (Ch.11)
uterine myoma 子宮筋腫 (Ch.11)
uterus 子宮 (Ch.7)
vagina 腟 (Ch.7)
valuables 貴重品 (Ch.16)
valve 弁 (Ch.7)
varicella 水痘 (Ch.11)
vein 静脈 (Ch.7)
vermiform appendix 虫垂 (Ch.6)
verruca いぼ (Ch.10)
vertebra 脊椎骨 (Ch.8)
visiting hours 面会時間 (Ch.17)
visitor 面会者 (Ch.2)
voice box 喉頭 (Ch.6)
vomit 吐く (Ch.13)
wait 待つ，*keep* 〜 *waiting* 〜を待たせておく (Ch.17)
walker 歩行器 (Ch.3)
wart いぼ (Ch.10)
washbasin 洗面器 (Ch.3)
weight scale 体重計 (Ch.3)
wheelchair 車椅子 (Ch.3)
white blood cell 白血球 (Ch.7)
whooping cough 百日咳 (Ch.11)
windpipe 気管 (Ch.6)
womb 子宮 (Ch.7)
work （薬などが）効く (Ch.16)
worry 心配する，気にする (Ch.13, 18)
worst 一番大変なところ，最も悪いこと (Ch.18)
wound 創傷，傷 (Ch.12)
wrist 手関節，手首 (Ch.5)
wrist bone 手根骨 (Ch.8)
X-ray technician 放射線技師 (Ch.2)
yeast infection カンジダ症 (Ch.11)

Index

和 英
(Ch.=Chapter)

青白い　pale（Ch.18）
あご　jaw（Ch.5）
汗をかく　perspire, sweat（Ch.13）
熱い　hot（Ch.13）
アレルギー　allergy（Ch.14）
アレルギーの　allergic（Ch.14）
慌てる　panic（Ch.18）
安全な　safe（Ch.16）
胃　stomach（Ch.6）
医院　clinic（Ch.17）
胃炎　gastritis, stomach ache（Ch.9）
胃潰瘍　stomach ulcer（Ch.9）
胃カメラ　gastroscope（Ch.3）
息　breath（Ch.15）
息切れ　short of breath（Ch.13）
息をする　breathe（Ch.13）
医師　doctor, physician, practitioner（Ch.1, 2, 16）
意識不明　unconscious（Ch.12）
痛い　painful, sore（Ch.12, 16）
痛み　pain（Ch.17）
痛む　hurt（Ch.13）
1日1回　once a day, quaque die (q.d.)（Ch.4）
一番大変なところ　worst（Ch.18）
（〜と）一緒にいる　stay (with 〜)（Ch.16, 18）
衣服　clothes（Ch.16）
いぼ　verruca, wart（Ch.10）
いる　stay（Ch.16, 18）
入れている　contain（Ch.16）
陰茎　penis（Ch.7）
咽喉　throat（Ch.6）
咽頭　pharynx（Ch.6）
うがい薬　gargle, mouthwash（Ch.4）
受付係　receptionist（Ch.2）
動かないでいる　hold still（Ch.15）
う蝕　cavity, dental caries（Ch.9）
うつ病　clinical depression（Ch.10）
うつ伏せになる　roll over onto one's stomach（Ch.15）
移る（移す）　transfer（Ch.16）
腕　arm（Ch.15）
うまく　great（Ch.18）
上着　shirt（Ch.15）
運動する　exercise（Ch.14）
栄養士　dietitian, nutritionist（Ch.2）

腋窩　armpit, axilla（Ch.5）
横隔膜　diaphragm（Ch.6）
黄疸　jaundice（Ch.11）
大きな病気　serious illness（Ch.14）
起き上がる　sit up（Ch.15）
教える　explain（Ch.16）
押す　press（Ch.17）
お大事に　take care of yourself（Ch.18）
頤　chin（Ch.5）
お風呂　bath（Ch.17）
重い病気　serious illness（Ch.14）
ガーゼ　gauze（Ch.3）
カート　cart（Ch.17）
会計窓口係　cashier（Ch.2）
介護福祉士　care giver, care worker（Ch.2）
外来患者　outpatient（Ch.2）
返す　return（Ch.17）
変える　change（Ch.16）
下顎骨　lower jaw, mandible（Ch.8）
額　forehead（Ch.5）
かぜ　common cold（Ch.9）
肩　shoulder（Ch.5）
花粉症　hay fever, pollinosis（Ch.9）
かゆい　itchy（Ch.13）
かわいた咳　dry cough（Ch.13）
肝炎　hepatitis（Ch.9）
眼科　ophthalmology（Ch.1）
眼科医　eye doctor, ophthalmologist（Ch.1）
肝硬変　cirrhosis of the liver, hepatic cirrhosis（Ch.9）
看護師　registered nurse (RN)（Ch.2）
カンジダ症　candidiasis, yeast infection（Ch.11）
感じる　feel（Ch.18）
関節　joint（Ch.8）
関節炎　arthritis（Ch.10）
感染症　infectious disease（Ch.10）
肝臓　liver（Ch.6）
含そう剤　gargle, mouthwash（Ch.4）
完璧な　perfect（Ch.18）
感冒　common cold（Ch.9）
漢方薬　herbal medicine（Ch.4）
気管　trachea, windpipe（Ch.6）
気管支炎　bronchitis（Ch.9）
効く（薬などが）　work（Ch.16）
傷　cut, wound（Ch.12）
傷跡　scar（Ch.12）
規則正しい　regular（Ch.14）
規則正しく　regularly（Ch.14）
貴重品　valuables（Ch.16）
気にする　worry（Ch.13, 18）
ギプス　cast（Ch.3）

気分（ここち）を感じる　feel（Ch.18）
休憩　break, rest（Ch.17, 18）
急性灰白髄炎　acute poliomyelitis（Ch.11）
吸入器　inhaler（Ch.3）
救命救急士　EMT (Emergency Medical Technician)（Ch.2）
胸骨　breastbone, sternum（Ch.8）
頬部　cheek（Ch.5）
胸部　chest（Ch.5）
胸部X線　chest X-ray（Ch.15）
緊張している　nervous（Ch.16）
筋肉　muscle（Ch.8）
くしゃみの発作　sneezing fits（Ch.13）
薬　medication, medicine（Ch.14, 16, 17）
首　neck（Ch.5）
繰り返して言う　repeat（Ch.17）
車椅子　wheelchair（Ch.3）
脛骨　shin bone, tibia（Ch.8）
形成外科　plastic surgery, reconstructive surgery（Ch.1）
形成外科医　plastic surgeon（Ch.1）
携帯電話　cellular phone（Ch.17）
頚部　neck（Ch.5）
痙攣　seizure（Ch.12）
けが　injury（Ch.12）
下剤　laxative（Ch.4）
血圧　blood pressure（Ch.15）
血圧計　blood pressure gauge, manometer, sphygmomanometer（Ch.3）
血液検体　blood sample, *take a blood sample* 採血する（Ch.15）
結核　tuberculosis (TB)（Ch.9）
月経過多　heavy menstrual periods, menorrhagia（Ch.11）
結婚する　marry（Ch.14）
欠如　absence（Ch.11）
血漿　plasma（Ch.7）
結腸　colon（Ch.6）
結膜炎　conjunctivitis, pink eye（Ch.11）
下痢　diarrhea, the runs（Ch.13）
腱　tendon（Ch.8）
肩甲骨　scapula, shoulder blade（Ch.8）
言語・音声障害　muteness（Ch.9）
検査　test（Ch.16）
検査結果　test results（Ch.16）
検査室　examination room（Ch.15）
研修医　clinical resident, resident（Ch.2）
抗菌薬　antibiotic(s)（Ch.4）
高血圧　high blood pressure (HBP), hypertension（Ch.10）
高脂血症　high blood fat, hyperlipidemia（Ch.10）
甲状腺　thyroid gland（Ch.7）
抗生物質　antibiotic(s)（Ch.4）

120

Index

喉頭　larynx, voice box（Ch.6）
喉頭炎　laryngitis（Ch.9）
更年期障害　menopausal disorder（Ch.11）
股関節部　hip（Ch.5）
呼吸器内科　pulmonology（Ch.1）
呼吸器内科医　pulmonologist（Ch.1）
試み　try（Ch.18）
個室　private room（Ch.16）
腰周り　hip（Ch.5）
骨　bone（Ch.8）
骨髄　bone marrow（Ch.7）
骨折　broken bone, fracture（Ch.12）
骨盤　pelvis（Ch.8）
鼓膜　eardrum, tympanic membrane（Ch.6）
こむら返り　cramp（Ch.12）
昏睡状態　coma（Ch.12）
昏睡状態の　comatose（Ch.12）
困難な　difficult（Ch.18）
採血する　take a blood sample（Ch.15）
最終月経　last period（Ch.14）
鎖骨　clavicle, collar bone（Ch.8）
擦過傷　scrape（Ch.12）
サプリメント　supplement（Ch.14）
妨げる　disturb（Ch.17）
坐薬　suppository（Ch.4）
産科　obstetrics（Ch.1）
産科医　obstetrician（Ch.1）
三角巾　sling（Ch.3）
産後うつ病　post-partum depression（Ch.11）
散剤　powdered medicine（Ch.4）
歯科　dentistry（Ch.1）
歯科医　dentist（Ch.1）
歯科衛生士　dental hygienist（Ch.2）
痔核　hemorrhoids, piles（Ch.9）
視覚障害　blindness（Ch.9）
子宮　uterus, womb（Ch.7）
子宮外妊娠　ectopic pregnancy, extrauterine pregnancy（Ch.11）
子宮筋腫　uterine fibroids, uterine myoma（Ch.11）
子宮頚管　cervix（Ch.7）
子宮頚がん　cervical cancer（Ch.11）
しこり　lump（Ch.12）
自殺　suicide（Ch.12）
自殺を図る　attempt suicide（Ch.12）
舌　tongue（Ch.6）
膝　knee（Ch.5）
耳痛　earache（Ch.13）
膝蓋骨　kneecap, patella（Ch.8）
じっとしている　hold still（Ch.15）
質問　question（Ch.17）
歯肉　gingiva, gum（Ch.6）
市販薬　over-the-counter medicine（OTC medicine）（Ch.4）
耳鼻咽喉科　otolaryngology, otorhinolaryngology（Ch.1）
耳鼻咽喉科医　ENT(Ear, Nose and Throat) doctor, otolaryngologist, otorhinolaryngologist（Ch.1）
自分自身　myself, *I haven't been myself lately.* 調子が悪い（Ch.13）
自閉症　autism（Ch.10）
シャツ　shirt（Ch.15）
尺骨　ulna（Ch.8）
じゃまをする　disturb（Ch.17）
シャワー　shower（Ch.16）
周期（月経などの）　period（Ch.13）
就寝時前　at bedtime, hora somni (h.s.)（Ch.4）
手関節　wrist（Ch.5）
手根骨　carpus, wrist bone（Ch.8）
主治医　attending physician（Ch.2）
手術　operation, surgery（Ch.4, 16）
手術室看護師　scrub nurse, surgical nurse（Ch.2）
腫瘍内科　oncology（Ch.1）
腫瘍内科医　oncologist（Ch.1）
腫瘤　lump（Ch.12）
循環器内科　cardiology（Ch.1）
循環器内科医　cardiologist（Ch.1）
消化器内科　gastroenterology（Ch.1）
消化器内科医　gastroenterologist（Ch.1）
上顎骨　maxilla, upper jaw（Ch.8）
錠剤　pill（Ch.4）
じょうずな　great（Ch.18）
使用説明　directions（Ch.4）
小腸　small intestine（Ch.6）
消毒液　disinfectant（Ch.3）
小児科　pediatrics（Ch.1）
小児科医　children's doctor, pediatrician（Ch.1）
踵部　heel（Ch.5）
静脈　vein（Ch.7）
上腕骨　humerus（Ch.8）
上腕部　upper arm（Ch.5）
職業　job, occupation（Ch.14）
食後　after meals, post cibum (p.c.)（Ch.4）
食事　meal（Ch.16, 17）
食中毒　food poisoning（Ch.9）
食道　esophagus（Ch.6）
食欲　appetite（Ch.14）
助産師　midwife（Ch.2）
処置台　treatment table（Ch.3）
処方する　prescribe（Ch.4）
処方せん　prescription（Ch.4）
尻　buttocks（Ch.5）
心筋梗塞　myocardial infarction (MI)（Ch.10）
神経　nerve（Ch.6）
神経症　neurosis（Ch.10）
神経内科　neurology（Ch.1）
神経内科医　neurologist（Ch.1）
人工呼吸　artificial respiration（Ch.12）
人工呼吸器　respirator（Ch.3）
人工透析　dialysis（Ch.4）
心臓　heart（Ch.7）
腎臓　kidney（Ch.7）
心臓病　heart problem（Ch.14）
心臓発作　heart attack（Ch.10）
靭帯　ligament（Ch.8）
身長計　height scale, scale（Ch.3）
陣痛　contractions, labor pains（Ch.11）
心配事　concern（Ch.17）
心配する　worry（Ch.13, 18）
心肺蘇生法　cardiopulmonary resuscitation (CPR)（Ch.12）
心配な　nervous（Ch.16）
腎不全　kidney failure, renal failure（Ch.10）
診療所　clinic（Ch.17）
膵臓　pancreas（Ch.6）
水痘　chickenpox, varicella（Ch.11）
水疱　blister（Ch.12）
髄膜炎　meningitis（Ch.9）
睡眠　rest（Ch.17, 18）
睡眠剤　sleeping pill（Ch.4）
頭蓋骨　cranium, skull（Ch.8）
ずきずきする（頭痛）　pounding (headache)（Ch.13）
ストレス　stress（Ch.14）
ストレッチャー　stretcher（Ch.3）
すばらしい　fine（Ch.18）
すまないと思う　sorry（Ch.17）
性感染症　sexually transmitted disease (STD)（Ch.10）
整形外科　orthopedics（Ch.1）
整形外科医　orthopedist（Ch.1）
精子　sperm（Ch.7）
生殖器　genitals（Ch.5）
精神科　psychiatrics（Ch.1）
精神科医　psychiatrist（Ch.1）
精巣　testicle（Ch.7）
脊髄　spinal cord（Ch.6）
脊椎（脊柱）　backbone, spine（Ch.8）
脊椎骨　vertebra（Ch.8）
舌　tongue（Ch.6）
舌圧子　tongue depressor（Ch.3）
赤血球　erythrocyte, red blood cell（Ch.7）
説明する　explain（Ch.16）
世話　care（Ch.18）
前額部　forehead（Ch.5）
喘息　asthma（Ch.9）

Supplement

洗面器	sink, washbasin (Ch.3)
洗面用具	toiletry (Ch.17)
前立腺	prostate (Ch.7)
前立腺肥大症	enlarged prostate, prostatomegaly (Ch.10)
前腕部	forearm (Ch.5)
臓器移植	organ transplantation (Ch.4)
創傷	cut, wound (Ch.12)
蒼白な	pale (Ch.18)
足関節	ankle (Ch.5)
足白癬	athlete's foot, fungal infection (Ch.10)
袖	sleeve (Ch.15)
(〜の)そばにいる	stay (with 〜) (Ch.16, 18)
退院する	check out (Ch.16)
退院手続き	check out procedures (Ch.16)
体温計	thermometer (Ch.15)
体重計	weight scale, scale (Ch.3)
大腿骨	femur, thigh bone (Ch.8)
大腿部	thigh (Ch.5)
大腸	large intestine (Ch.6)
胎盤	placenta (Ch.7)
ダウン症候群	Down syndrome (Ch.10)
タオル	towel (Ch.17)
立ちくらみがする	dizzy (Ch.13)
脱臼	dislocation (Ch.12)
タバコ	cigarette (Ch.14)
タバコを吸う	smoke (Ch.14)
食べ物	food (Ch.17)
食べる	eat (Ch.17)
打撲傷	bruise (Ch.12)
だるい	dull, sluggish (Ch.13)
だるさ	fatigue (Ch.13)
痰	phlegm (Ch.13)
単純疱疹	herpes simplex (Ch.10)
担当看護師	primary nurse (Ch.17)
胆嚢	gallbladder (Ch.6)
痰を伴った咳	productive cough (Ch.13)
力をぬく	relax (Ch.15)
チクッと痛ませる	prick (Ch.15)
腟	vagina (Ch.7)
窒息	asphyxiation, suffocation (Ch.12)
注意欠陥多動性障害	attention deficit hyperactivity disorder (ADHD) (Ch.11)
中耳炎	middle ear infection, otitis media (Ch.9)
注射器	syringe (Ch.3)
虫垂	appendix, vermiform appendix (Ch.6)
肘部	elbow (Ch.5)
腸	bowel, *regular bowel movements* 規則正しい便通 (Ch.14)
聴覚障害	deafness (Ch.9)
調子が悪い	dull, sluggish, I haven't been myself (Ch.13)
聴診器	stethoscope (Ch.3)
直腸	rectum (Ch.6)
鎮咳剤	cough medicine, cough suppressant (Ch.4)
鎮痛剤	analgesic, painkiller (Ch.4)
痛風	gout (Ch.10)
使う	use (Ch.17)
疲れ	fatigue (Ch.13)
疲れ(させる)	tire (Ch.13)
続ける	keep (going) (Ch.18)
つま先	hallux, toe (Ch.5)
詰まっている(鼻などが)	stuffed up (Ch.13)
詰まらせる	choke (Ch.12)
爪	nail (Ch.5)
つらい	difficult (Ch.18)
つわり	nausea and vomiting during pregnancy (NVP), morning sickness (Ch.11)
手	arm (Ch.15)
T-シャツ	t-shirt (Ch.15)
定期的に	regularly (Ch.14)
低体温	hypothermia (Ch.12)
溺水する	drown (Ch.12)
手首	wrist (Ch.5)
手伝う	help (Ch.18)
手続き	procedure (Ch.16, 17)
点滴	IV (intravenous) (Ch.16)
点滴静脈注射	IV drip (Ch.4)
点滴スタンド	IV stand (Ch.3)
点滴棒	IV pole (Ch.3)
殿部	buttocks (Ch.5)
橈骨	radius (Ch.8)
糖尿病	diabetes, diabetes mellitus (DM) (Ch.9)
動脈硬化症	arteriosclerosis (Ch.10)
動脈	artery (Ch.7)
動脈硬化症	hardening of the arteries (Ch.10)
投薬量	dosage, dose (Ch.4)
とどまる	stay (Ch.16, 18)
止まらないくしゃみ	sneezing fits (Ch.13)
努力	try (Ch.18)
トレイ	tray (Ch.17)
ナースコールボタン	call button (Ch.17)
内科	internal medicine (Ch.1)
内科医	internist, physician (Ch.1, 2)
ないこと	absence (Ch.11)
内視鏡	endoscope (Ch.3)
内分泌科	endocrinology (Ch.1)
内分泌科医	endocrinologist (Ch.1)
軟膏	salve, ointment (Ch.4)
軟骨	cartilage (Ch.8)
にきび	acne, acne vulgaris (Ch.10)
握りこぶし	fist (Ch.15)
肉	meat (Ch.16)
入院患者	inpatient (Ch.2)
入院させる	hospitalize (Ch.14)
乳がん	breast cancer (Ch.11)
乳頭	nipple (Ch.5)
乳房	breast (Ch.5)
乳幼児突然死症候群	sudden infant death syndrome (SIDS) (Ch.11)
尿	urine (Ch.7)
尿管	ureter (Ch.7)
尿検体	urine sample (Ch.15)
尿道	urethra (Ch.7)
尿路感染症	urinary tract infection (UTI) (Ch.10)
妊娠悪阻	nausea and vomiting during pregnancy (NVP), morning sickness (Ch.11)
認知症	dementia, senility (Ch.10)
寝返りをうつ	roll over, *roll over onto one's stomach* うつ伏せになる (Ch.15)
熱	fever (Ch.14)
熱傷	burn (Ch.12)
熱中症	heat stroke, sunstroke (Ch.10)
熱っぽい	feverish (Ch.13)
眠る	sleep (Ch.13)
捻挫	sprain (Ch.12)
脳	brain (Ch.6)
脳神経外科	neurosurgery (Ch.1)
脳神経外科医	neurosurgeon (Ch.1)
脳しんとう	concussion (Ch.12)
脳卒中	cerebrovascular accident (CVA), stroke (Ch.9)
喉が渇いている	thirsty (Ch.13)
肺	lung (Ch.6)
肺炎	pneumonia (Ch.9)
肺がん	lung carcinoma, lung cancer (Ch.9)
排尿する	urinate (Ch.14)
吐き気がする	nauseous (Ch.13)
吐く	vomit (Ch.13)
白血球	leukocyte, white blood cell (Ch.7)
白血病	leukemia (Ch.9)
話す	speak (Ch.17)
鼻水	runny nose (Ch.13)
速くなる(脈などが)	race (Ch.13)
針	needle (Ch.3)
鼻腔	nasal cavity (Ch.6)
腓骨	fibula (Ch.8)
尾骨	coccyx, tail bone (Ch.8)
膝	knee (Ch.5)
肘	elbow (Ch.5)
脾臓	spleen (Ch.7)

Index

泌尿器科　urology　(Ch.1)
泌尿器科医　urologist　(Ch.1)
避妊薬　contraceptive　(Ch.4)
皮膚　skin　(Ch.5)
皮膚科　dermatology　(Ch.1)
皮膚科医　dermatologist, skin doctor　(Ch.1)
肥満　obesity　(Ch.10)
百日咳　pertussis, whooping cough　(Ch.11)
病院　hospital　(Ch.17)
病棟師長　head nurse　(Ch.2)
貧血　anemia　(Ch.9)
不安な　nervous　(Ch.16)
風疹　German measles, rubella　(Ch.11)
不快な感じ　discomfort　(Ch.17)
副作用　side effect　(Ch.16)
腹部　abdomen　(Ch.5)
含む　contain　(Ch.16)
婦人科　gynecology　(Ch.1)
婦人科医　gynecologist　(Ch.1)
豚肉　pork　(Ch.16)
不眠症　insomnia　(Ch.10)
ブラジャー　bra　(Ch.15)
風呂　bath　(Ch.17)
分娩　delivery　(Ch.11)
便　feces, stool　(Ch.6)
弁　valve　(Ch.7)
便器　bedpan　(Ch.3)
返却する　return　(Ch.17)
片頭痛　migraine　(Ch.9)
便通　*regular bowel movements*　規則正しい便通　(Ch.14)
扁桃腺　tonsil　(Ch.6)
便秘をさせる　constipate　(Ch.13)
縫合　stitches, sutures　(Ch.3)

膀胱　bladder, urinary bladder　(Ch.7)
膀胱炎　cystitis　(Ch.11)
放射線科　radiology　(Ch.1)
放射線科医　radiologist　(Ch.1)
放射線技師　X-ray technician　(Ch.2)
疱疹　cold sore　(Ch.10)
包帯　bandage　(Ch.3)
頬　cheek　(Ch.5)
保健師　community health nurse　(Ch.2)
保険証　health insurance card　(Ch.17)
保護　care　(Ch.18)
歩行器　walker　(Ch.3)
保護者　guardian　(Ch.2)
補聴器　hearing aid　(Ch.3)
発疹　rash　(Ch.13)
骨　bone　(Ch.8)
ポリオ　polio　(Ch.11)
まくる（袖などを）　roll up　(Ch.15)
麻疹　measles, rubeola　(Ch.11)
麻酔科医　anesthesiologist　(Ch.1)
麻酔科　anesthesiology　(Ch.1)
（〜を）待たせておく　keep 〜 waiting　(Ch.17)
待つ　wait　(Ch.17)
松葉杖　crutch　(Ch.3)
麻痺　paralysis　(Ch.12)
慢性疾患　chronic illness　(Ch.10, 14)
水薬　liquid medicine　(Ch.4)
水虫　athlete's foot, fungal infection　(Ch.10)
耳の痛み　earache　(Ch.13)
［脈などが］速くなる　race　(Ch.13)
眠前　at bedtime, hora somni (h.s.)　(Ch.4)
無月経　absence of periods, amenorrhea　(Ch.11)

虫歯　cavity, dental caries　(Ch.9)
目が覚めている　awake　(Ch.16)
めまいがする　dizzy　(Ch.13)
面会時間　visiting hours　(Ch.17)
面会者　visitor　(Ch.2)
もう一度言ってください　Pardon me?　(Ch.17)
もう一度やってみる　give it another try　(Ch.18)
申し分ない　fine　(Ch.18)
最も悪いこと　worst　(Ch.18)
戻す　return　(Ch.17)
薬剤師　pharmacist　(Ch.2)
輸血　blood transfusion　(Ch.4)
ゆっくり　slowly　(Ch.15, 17)
横になる　lie down　(Ch.15, 18)
卵巣　ovary　(Ch.7)
卵巣がん　ovarian cancer　(Ch.11)
リウマチ　rheumatism　(Ch.10)
理解する　see, understand　(Ch.18)
理学療法士　physical therapist　(Ch.2)
流行性耳下腺炎　mumps, parotitis　(Ch.11)
流産　miscarriage, spontaneous abortion　(Ch.11)
臨床心理士　clinical psychologist　(Ch.2)
リンパ節　lymph node　(Ch.7)
裂傷　laceration　(Ch.12)
老年内科　geriatrics　(Ch.1)
老年内科医　geriatrician　(Ch.1)
肋骨　rib　(Ch.8)
わかる　see, understand　(Ch.18)
割れそうな（頭痛）　splitting (headache)　(Ch.13)

memo

memo

Acknowledgments

Completion of this book would not have been possible without the guidance, patience, and understanding of our editor, Katsuji Koeda, and the staff at Nanzando. Thanks must also go to the anonymous reviewer of the first draft, for identifying and remedying many faults in the word lists. We also thank Hideko Chujo and Miki Morita for producing countless copies of early drafts. Thanks are extended to Masayo Toume and Kimie Tanimoto of the School of Nursing, Kagawa University, for their advice when this project was at an early stage. Thanks are also due to Yukari Willey and Shin Segawa for their advice and support throughout this demanding project.

Finally, we thank the faculty, staff, and students of the Faculty of Medicine, Kagawa University, to whom this book is dedicated.

謝　辞

この書を完成するにあたり，南山堂 編集部 小枝克寿氏はじめ，スタッフ諸氏の指導と協力，忍耐と理解に深く感謝する．また，ドラフトの段階から語彙リストの誤字，誤植等を指摘し修正いただいた多くの方々にも感謝したい．中条ヒデ子，森田美樹両氏には，幾度となる初期のドラフトを複写し協力いただいた．香川大学看護学科 當目雅代氏，谷本公重氏にも，この企画の初期の段階において助言を受けた．さらに，この難しいプロジェクトに支援と助言を与えていただいたウィリーゆかり氏と勢川 慎氏にも同等の感謝の気持ちを表したい．

最後に，香川大学医学部の教員，事務，学生諸氏に感謝するとともに，この本を捧げたい．

看単! Easy Nursing English

2009 年 2 月 12 日　1 版 1 刷　　　　　　　　　© 2009
2020 年 7 月 31 日　　　　　5 刷

著　者
Ian Willey　　Gerardine McCrohan　　芝田征二

発行者
株式会社 南山堂　代表者 鈴木幹太
〒113-0034　東京都文京区湯島 4-1-11
TEL 代表 03-5689-7850　　www.nanzando.com

ISBN 978-4-525-02231-0　　定価（本体 1,200 円＋税）

JCOPY ＜出版者著作権管理機構 委託出版物＞
複製を行う場合はそのつど事前に（一社）出版者著作権管理機構（電話03-5244-5088, FAX 03-5244-5089, e-mail: info@jcopy.or.jp）の許諾を得るようお願いいたします.

本書の内容を無断で複製することは，著作権法上での例外を除き禁じられています．また，代行業者等の第三者に依頼してスキャニング，デジタルデータ化を行うことは認められておりません．

―本書をお使いの先生方へ―

補足教材
「Easy Quizzes」
「Easy Reviews & Easy Exams」
「Easy Speaking & Writing Tasks」
南山堂のサイトで配布しています．

www.nanzando.com
「看単！Easy Nursing English」の
ページをご覧ください．